THE EPILEPSY REFERENCE BOOK

THE EPILEPSY REFERENCE BOOK

Direct and Clear Answers to Everyone's Questions

by
Peter M Jeavons, Hon D.Sc., FRCP, FRCPsych
Visiting Professor, Clinical Neurophysiology Unit
University of Aston in Birmingham
and
Alec Aspinall
Senior Regional Officer and Director of Education
British Epilepsy Association

Harper & Row, Publishers
London

Cambridge
Hagerstown
Philadelphia
New York

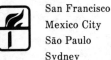

San Francisco
Mexico City
São Paulo
Sydney

Copyright © 1985 Peter M Jeavons & Alec Aspinall
First published 1985 reprinted 1985 (twice)
All rights reserved

Harper & Row Ltd
28 Tavistock Street
London WC2E 7PN

British Library Cataloguing in Publication Data

Jeavons, Peter M.
    The epilepsy reference book.
    1. Epilepsy
    I. Title   II. Aspinall, Alec
    616.8'53   RC372

    ISBN 0-06-318312-9

Typeset by Burns & Smith, Derby
Printed and bound by Butler and Tanner, Frome and London

This book is dedicated with affection
to our friends Maurice Parsonage and George Burden
who have done so much to help all those who have epilepsy.

Contents

ACKNOWLEDGEMENTS

This book could not have been written without the help of many colleagues who responded so readily when we asked them to send us a list of questions. We are particularly grateful to: Tim Betts; Brian Bower; Neil Cartlidge; Jean Cheetham; Michael Espir; Brian Gibberd; Richard Grant; Harry Hayward; Derek Howe; Ivan MacIntyre; Ian McKinlay; Jolyon Oxley; Maurice Parsonage; Ron Radley; Euan Ross; Michael Saunders; Greg Stores.

We have been encouraged in our task by the interest shown in the book by the British Epilepsy Association. We are greatly indebted to our secretaries Margaret Geddes and Joan Watton for typing the questions and answers and to Margaret for typing the final draft.

Finally, our thanks go to all those who actually asked the questions and we hope we have helped them.

INTRODUCTION

This book is not a textbook but is designed for those who have specific questions to ask about epilepsy — people who themselves are prone to this condition and their families; members of the medical and nursing professions whose task it is to help the epileptic person; social workers, teachers, employers and others for whom an understanding of epilepsy is essential.

Its aim is to provide in simple language answers to questions that are commonly asked about the nature of epilepsy and seizures, methods of treatment, education, employment and problems of living with epilespy.

In the past, patients were not encouraged to ask their doctor questions about their illness, its treatment and management. Although the attitude of the medical profession has changed, many patients are still nervous or unwilling to ask their doctor questions, whether he be in hospital or in general practice. If the patient (or parent) is to cope with any illness, it is essential to have a knowledge of the facts. It is not always easy to answer a simple question in a simple way, and there may be several answers to many questions, depending upon the opinion of the 'expert'. In this book, where opinions of the experts differ, the answers have been based on the various views.

The questions throughout the book are only those that have been asked by patients or parents or relatives. They have been collected from our colleagues, doctors, teachers and social workers who have a special interest in epilepsy, and also from the files of the British Epilepsy Association. If a subject is omitted it is because no one has asked about it, or perhaps it has only been asked by one person.

All statistics about epilepsy can be misleading, for several main reasons:

1 People conceal the fact that they or their relatives have epilepsy and there is often a lack of accurate information about family history.
2 Probably about one-fifth of people said to have epilepsy do not have it.
3 Some people have epilepsy which has not been diagnosed — no one has suggested how common this is.
4 Information about epilepsy comes from doctors who work in hospitals or special centres, or from other people who are dealing with the problems of people with epilepsy. This must give an artificial bias to the picture, since there is less information about people who have no problems when they have epilepsy.
5 Definitions of seizures are often inadequate or inaccurate and there is no proper classification.

Finally, it is very important to realize that the questions in this book have come from people who have sought advice about their epilepsy. This means that many of them have had some problems because they have epilepsy. However, there are many people who have no problems at all.

To the reader

This book is based on the actual questions that people have asked. You may need information about particular topics. Select the topics that most concern you and you may be surprised to find that other people ask the same questions as you. The index below indicates question numbers.

1 Seizures: 1 to 13, 17, 20 to 22, 25, 40, 41, 59, 61, 65, 70 to 74
2 Causes of epilepsy: 26 to 39, 42 to 48, 51 to 56, 58

1

Epilepsy

The brain is made up of millions of tiny nerve cells called neurones. The function of the brain is to tell us about our surroundings, and the brain controls our body and all our actions, our thoughts, our awareness and our memory. Information is sent to the brain through sense organs of sight, sound, smell, taste and touch.

Each brain cell can receive and send messages in a very similar way to the simple units that make up calculators and computers. Thus the cell can accept or refuse a message and can send it on to another cell. The cell can be switched on or off. Some messages tell other cells to act (activation), some messages stop other cells acting (inhibition).

The nerve cell consists of a body with a long arm, the axon, which sends messages, and short arms, called dendrites, which receive messages (Figure 1.1). One cell may connect with several other cells and may receive messages from several cells. Although electrical changes occur in the cells, the messages from one cell to another are transmitted by various chemicals (neurotransmitters).

Normally, messages are sent and received in an orderly way. If brain cells start acting on their own, or pass messages that they should not pass, or do not respond to messages, an epileptic seizure may result. All cells are then acting in an unusual way, so something unusual will happen. What happens will depend on where the abnormal activity occurs, and whether it spreads to other parts of the brain.

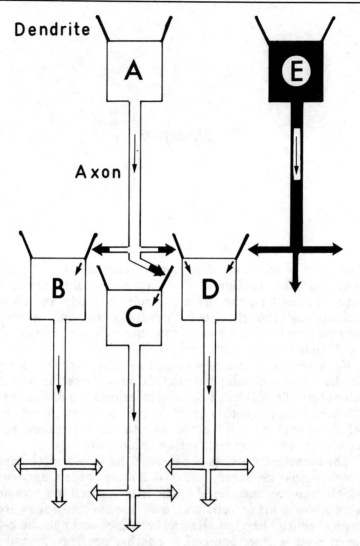

Figure 1.1 Messages from cell A are sent down the axon to the dendrites of cells B, C and D. The message from A tells B, C and D to act, and to pass on messages to other cells (activation). Messages from cell E are sent to the dendrite of cell D, telling cell D *not* to act (inhibition).

If the epileptic discharge involves the whole brain from the start, the seizure is called primary generalized. When the discharge affects only part of the brain, the result is a partial seizure. Sometimes the discharge spreads from part of the brain to involve the whole brain, an attack is then called a partial seizure with secondary generalization.

Figure 1.2 shows a view of half of the brain seen from the side. The various parts of the brain have different functions. Messages to and from the right side of the body go to the left half of the brain and vice versa. The occipital lobe is concerned with vision, the parietal lobe with sensation and the motor cortex in the frontal lobe with movement. All areas communicate with other areas, but the temporal lobe is particularly concerned with sorting out messages from other parts of the brain, and is the storehouse for memory.

The exact nature of the partial seizure depends on the localized area of the brain involved. Thus, a discharge that occurs in that part of the motor cortex (this is the covering of the brain containing the brain cells) responsible for movements of the thumb will result in the thumb jerking. If the discharge occurs in the part of the sensory cortex that receives messages from the foot, a sensation will be felt as if it were coming from the foot. As long as the discharge only occurs in one part of the brain, the person remains conscious and is aware of something peculiar happening to his body. Sometimes the abnormal movement or sensation continues for a minute or so and then stops. This is called a simple partial seizure. Another name is a focal seizure.

If the discharge lasts a few seconds and then rapidly spreads to involve the whole brain, becoming generalized, the first part of the seizure is called an aura. An aura is something experienced by a person with epilepsy and is a warning that a loss of consciousness or a generalized seizure may occur. It is the start of a seizure. An aura is very short, lasting seconds, very rarely minutes. When someone has a severe tonic-clonic seizure, he often does not remember the first few moments of the seizure, so afterwards he may have forgotten that he had an aura. If drug treatment makes a tonic-clonic seizure shorter and less severe, the person may then remember what happened at the start, and think that

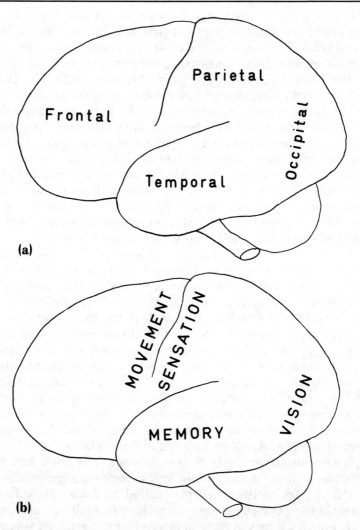

Figure 1.2 Side view of the brain, showing the main lobes (a) and the areas involved in various activities (b). The frontal and parietal lobes are separated by the Rolandic fissure, and the temporal and parietal lobes are separated by the Sylvian fissure. The occipital lobe is at the back of the brain and below it is the cerebellum.

the pattern of the seizure has changed because he now has an aura.

Seizures used to be divided into two sorts — grand-mal or major seizures and petit-mal or minor seizures — but these two terms are not accurate, especially petit-mal which included a lot of different types of seizure. Seizures have therefore now been renamed (see p. 10).

Grand-mal or major seizures are now called tonic-clonic seizures. Although a tonic-clonic seizure may be frightening to see, especially on the first occasion, there is a simple explanation for its various features.

Firstly, activity often ceases for a few seconds and the person may stare. Then the muscles contract — this is the tonic phase. Because the muscles of the back that keep us upright tend to be stronger than those that cause us to bend forward, the body tends to arch and fall backwards. The muscles of the chest wall contract forcing air out of the lungs through the vocal chords in the throat and, since these have also contracted, a high-pitched sound or a cry may occur. Next all the muscles start jerking and this is the clonic phase. Increased saliva is produced in the mouth and may dribble out (this is the so-called 'foaming'). The contractions of the jaw muscles may further damage the tongue or cheek. During all this time the person is not breathing, and so will become blue or purple. Sometimes contraction of the bladder and stomach wall may result in the passing of urine or, very rarely, of faeces.

Once the brain cells are exhausted, the movements cease and the person will take extra deep breaths to restore the oxygen supply to the brain. This heavy breathing is often noisy and is called stertorous breathing. Many people sleep after a tonic-clonic seizure and when they recover fully they often have a very severe headache and their muscles may ache.

If you need a more detailed explanation of how the brain works, read 'Epilepsy — the facts' by Anthony Hopkins (see p. 107).

Seizures

1 What is epilepsy?

Epilepsy is an established tendency to recurrent seizures. The seizure or fit is the result of an abnormal discharge of brain cells.

Anyone can have a seizure if exposed to a strong insult (an insult is any stimulus that the brain does not like, e.g. an electric current). The term epileptic threshold, or seizure or convulsive threshold, is used to describe the likelihood of any particular person having a seizure. People who have epilepsy are said to have a low seizure threshold, because they may have a seizure if the working of the brain is only slightly upset. Others are able to withstand quite a big insult to the brain without having a seizure and they have a high convulsive threshold. This threshold depends on the person's genes, which means it is inherited. People with a low convulsive threshold may show spike and wave in their electroencephalograph (EEG).

Spike and wave, at 3 cycles per second, is illustrated in Figure 1.3, which shows a long discharge associated with an absence. The spike and wave pattern is inherited, and various types of seizure may occur in association. Often the discharge lasts only a few seconds, and no seizure is apparent.

2 If you have one fit does this mean you have epilepsy?

If you have only one seizure this does not mean that you have epilepsy. By definition, epilepsy means that a person is likely to have recurring seizures.

3 How many different types of epileptic fit are there?

The word seizure is now more commonly used by doctors and is more widely accepted than the word 'fit'.

Many people think that only two sorts of seizure occur in epilepsy — 'grand-mal' and 'petit-mal'. Grand-mal seizures are called major fits, but the modern term is tonic-clonic seizures. The name has been changed because if someone

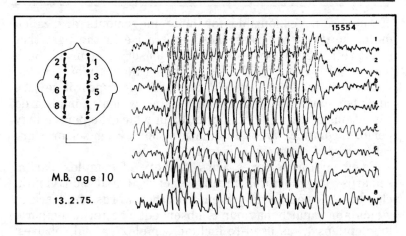

Figure 1.3 Spike and wave discharge in a girl aged 10 years. The discharge lasts 6 seconds and consists of bilateral spike and wave occurring three times every second, and occurring on both sides of the brain. During the discharge the child had an absence. The EEG is normal before and after the spike and wave discharge. (Reproduced from "Epilepsy Today — Electroencephalography." P M Jeavons, by kind permission of Geigy Pharmaceuticals.)

suddenly falls down, jerks once or twice, passes urine, but gets up after a few seconds, one should not call the attack a grand-mal (which is French for big illness), nor should one call it petit-mal (though it is a little illness), but it is a tonic-clonic seizure. Tonic means going stiff and clonic means jerking. Petit-mal should no longer be used because in the past it included absences, myoclonic jerks, brief tonic-clonic seizures and complex partial seizures; in other words any attack that was not a grand mal.

Seizures are divided into two main groups — those that are generalized from the start, involving both sides of the brain or the central regions, and those that involve only part of the brain (partial). In primary generalized epilepsy, seizures may be *tonic-clonic* (grand-mal, major fits), *myoclonic* (myo means muscle and clonic means jerk, so these are bilateral jerks of muscles) or *absences* (petit-mal).

Seizures arising from only part of the brain are called partial seizures or fits. Partial seizures that arise in that part of the brain responsible for body movements are called motor seizures, whereas those that arise in the part that interprets sensations are called sensory seizures. Both motor and sensory seizures can be called *simple partial seizures* (focal fits is the old term). These types of seizure contrast with partial seizures in which complicated sensations or experiences occur, or in which the person may perform complicated or automatic actions. Such seizures are called *complex partial seizures*.

Psychomotor seizures are a variety of complex partial seizures. Psychomotor means emotional and behavioural changes, as well as movement; in other words an attack in which abnormal behaviour is observed. The term temporal lobe epilepsy was used to include complex partial seizures, psychomotor seizures, and seizures in which there was an aura with complicated symptoms such as abnormalities of thought, awareness, memory, etc.

Seizures in children are often different from those in adults, and some sorts of seizure are only found at particular ages. Thus there are seizures that only happen in the first few weeks of life and these are called *neonatal* (newborn) seizures. *Febrile convulsions* (seizures in a child who has a high temperature) are likely to happen especially between the ages of 6 months and 3 years and are rarely seen after the age of 5 years. A rare form of epilepsy which starts in the first year of life is West Syndrome, in which the seizures are called *infantile spasms*. Somewhat similar attacks, in which there are jerks and often falls, occur in children between 1 and 4 years, and these attacks may be called *myoclonic and atonic* fits, and this is known as Lennox-Gastaut Syndrome.

Many of the partial seizures that start in childhood (usually after the age of 3 years) will disappear of their own accord around puberty and they are therefore called benign partial (or focal) epilepsies of childhood, and are named after the part of the brain involved (e.g. *benign Rolandic seizures* or *benign centro-temporal seizures*). Seizures in which the person's head turns to one side, and perhaps the whole body then turns in a circle, are called *versive or adversive* seizures. Other types of seizure occur but are rare.

12

4   Is it possible to have more than one type of fit?

Occasional tonic-clonic seizures may occur in people who have absences or myoclonic jerks. Tonic-clonic seizures may also occur in a person with partial seizures if the abnormal discharge that occurs in a localized area of the brain spreads to become generalized. Such a person could therefore have two types of seizure, a partial seizure or focal fit, and a secondary generalized tonic-clonic seizure.

Several types of seizure are common in severe myoclonic epilepsies of childhood (Lennox-Gastaut Syndrome), and in people where the epilepsy is a symptom of brain disease or disorder.

5   Is a fit the same thing as epilepsy?

A fit or seizure is the main symptom in epilepsy, but the words seizure and epilepsy are not the same. For example, in primary generalized *epilepsy*, the EEG may show spike and wave, a genetically determined pattern that indicates a low seizure threshold. In primary generalized epilepsy the types of *seizures* may be tonic-clonic, absences or myoclonic jerks.

6   What is the difference between a fit and a convulsion?

The term fit or seizure includes attacks in which there may be no movements of the body. A convulsion usually means that consciousness is lost and that there is jerking, and the word convulsion is often used to mean the same as a tonic-clonic seizure or major fit. All convulsions are seizures, but not all seizures are convulsions.

7   Am I epileptic or just having convulsions?

The word epileptic is often misused. It should be used as an adjective. Thus, a person who has epilepsy can have an epileptic seizure and anyone who has repeated convulsions has epilepsy. Such a person might object to being called 'an epileptic'. However, it does not appear to worry people with diabetes if they are called diabetics. Furthermore, an EEG abnormality cannot itself be epileptic, though it may indicate a tendency to epilepsy.

8   Are febrile convulsions epileptic?

A febrile convulsion is an epileptic fit or seizure. This does not mean that subsequent epilepsy will occur once the child has grown up. In the past there has been a tendency to avoid the word epilepsy when talking about febrile convulsions, and parents often say that their child has febrile convulsions but not epilepsy. Febrile convulsions are common in some families. At least 60% of children who have a febrile convulsion will never have another. It is very rare for epileptic attacks to continue later in the child's life and the child who has had a febrile convulsion probably only has a 4% chance of developing epilepsy.

9   What is petit-mal?

Petit-mal is French for small illness and it was a name given to all sorts of seizure that were not grand-mal (a big illness). Thus, petit-mal was used to describe absences, myoclonic jerks, brief complex partial seizures and short tonic-clonic seizures. The term petit-mal should not therefore be used unless it is clear that it means only an absence. Absences are always associated with 3 cycles per second spike and wave in the EEG.

There are two types of absence. In *simple absences* activity stops, the person stares and there are no movements, although occasionally very slight movements of the eyelids may occur. The seizure lasts less than 15 seconds, usually only 5 to 10 seconds, and at the end of the attack activity re-starts. In *complex absences* activity stops or may continue. Automatic actions are common and consist of aimless movements, smacking of the lips, sucking, making movements of the mouth, uttering some sound, touching the body, making slight movements of hands or arms. A complex absence often lasts longer than 15 seconds. It may be very difficult from observation only to distinguish complex absences from psychomotor seizures. Recovery after a complex absence is usually rapid and no confusion ensues, whereas some degree of confusion occurs after a psychomotor seizure. In complex absences the EEG shows spike and wave, in contrast to a focal abnormality in the psychomotor attacks.

10 What is a Jacksonian fit?

A Jacksonian fit is the name given to some focal motor fits, which are now called simple-partial seizures. Hughlings Jackson was a famous neurologist who described this sort of seizure. In some Jacksonian fits the symptoms start in one part of an arm or leg and then spread into other parts. This has been called a 'march of events', and is extremely rare.

11 Do people get a warning before they have a fit?

People with partial epilepsy may get a warning that they are going to have a tonic-clonic seizure. This warning is called an *aura*. It is not a warning that a fit will occur, but that consciousness may be lost. The aura is the start of the seizure. As long as the abnormal discharges in the brain are confined to only a part of the brain, the person remains conscious and may be aware of sensations or movements. Once the discharges spread to the centre of the brain consciousness is lost. The nature of the aura depends on the area of the brain in which the abnormal discharge occurs. An aura usually lasts only a few seconds. Some people will only get an aura if the abnormal discharge is very short and does not spread through the brain. If the tonic-clonic seizure is a severe one, after the attack the person may not remember anything about the few seconds before the loss of consciousness so may not be aware that they had an aura. If fits become shorter with treatment, the patient may now remember the warning and think that there has been a change in the pattern of their seizures.

Some people, especially those who have complex partial seizures, experience symptoms for some hours or even days before they have a fit. Such symptoms are not called aura, but are called prodromal symptoms, and may include headache, irritability, or upset stomach or gut etc.

12 How long does a fit last?

The length of a seizure depends on the type of seizure. Myoclonic jerks last a second or so, absences usually last 5–10 seconds or sometimes up to a minute. A tonic-clonic seizure lasts a few minutes, although recovery to full consciousness takes longer.

13   Does one become unconscious in every type of fit?

Complete loss of consciousness occurs in tonic-clonic seizures (major fits). In some minor fits like myoclonic jerks, there is no apparent loss of consciousness. In some seizures there may be loss of awareness, although the person does not lose consciousness altogether and may perform quite complicated actions. These complicated actions are known as automatisms.

14   Will people swallow their tongue?

In a tonic-clonic seizure, after the jerking movements stop, breathing will re-start. If the person is lying on his or her back, the tongue may fall backwards and this stops air going down the windpipe. In order to stop this happening, the person should be turned on to one side and a pillow or rolled up clothing should be placed under the head.

15   Foaming at the mouth is horrible to see. Does this mean that the person is mad?

In a tonic-clonic seizure there may be an increase in the amount of saliva in the mouth, so that it dribbles out. If the tongue or cheek has been bitten, this spittle may be blood-stained. Foaming at the mouth is a very old term and was used in the past because people thought that if a person had a fit they were mad. This is quite untrue. An increase in saliva may of course occur in other types of seizure, especially in complex-partial seizures.

In some countries, especially Africa and India, epilepsy is thought to be catching because of this frothing of the mouth, and people will avoid touching the person who has had a fit, or even walking over the ground where they lay. This idea is quite wrong, and epilepsy is neither infectious nor contagious.

16   Can ones speech be affected by a seizure?

Yes, if the abnormal discharge of brain cells occurs in that part of the brain responsible for speech. As a result, the person may be unable to speak, or their speech may be altered so that the words or sentences do not come out clearly or in a sensible or understandable way. Sometimes the person may say something distinctly, but what they say is not related to the circumstances.

17 What is meant by epileptic status?

Epileptic status means that one seizure is followed immediately by another without any period of recovery between. The most common and most dangerous type of status is that in which the repeated seizures are tonic-clonic. *Tonic-clonic status* is a medical emergency and needs immediate hospital admission because it can be fatal unless treated properly. It must be stressed that the diagnosis of tonic-clonic status only applies if the patient goes from one fit to another without any intervals, and it does not apply to someone who has many fits during one day, but who recovers, however briefly, between each one.

Minor status is not life-threatening. Frequent and continuous generalized jerking without loss of consciousness is called *myoclonic status*. *Absence status* is also called spike wave stupor and the patient behaves like a zombie. *Complex partial status* is rare; the patient is confused and behaviour is abnormal and there may be automatisms. *Simple partial status* usually involves jerking of part of the body which continues for hours or days, and the medical name of this is epilepsia partialis continua.

The EEG is often important in the differential diagnosis of epileptic status.

18 Do fits impair the memory?

Many people with epilepsy complain of a poor memory and there are many reasons for impairment of memory. Memory can be poor if the brain has been damaged, but it can also be poor for psychological reasons. Disturbances of memory are most common in people whose epilepsy is due to abnormality in the temporal lobe, because this part of the brain is most concerned with memory. Long seizures, very frequent seizures, very frequent discharges in the EEG of spikes or spike and wave may affect memory even if these discharges are very brief. In some cases memory may be affected by antiepileptic drugs, but this is a less common cause.

19 Do fits damage the brain?

Only if the tonic-clonic seizure (including febrile convulsions) is very long, lasting more than 15 minutes. During a long attack, which is really a status epilepticus, shortage of oxygen may damage part of the brain, especially the temporal lobe. This damage is more likely to occur in the young child, but a long status epilepticus in an adult can cause damage. Most seizures are too short to cause damage.

20 Can epilepsy happen at any age?

Seizures can start at any age and certain types of seizure appear to be related to age, starting at a particular time of life and often finishing by a certain age. Examples are febrile convulsions, which commonly appear between the ages of 6 months and 3 years and which disappear by the age of 5 or 6 years. Benign epilepsies of childhood start in early childhood and disappear around puberty. However, some seizures may start around puberty. Epilepsy starting much later in life may be a symptom of other disease, but not necessarily so.

21 Is there a particular point in ones life when fits are most likely to occur?

The appearance of some types of seizure depends on age. Thus, infantile spasms (West Syndrome) appear before the age of 1 year, myoclonic jerks may start around 3 years or later around puberty. Absences usually start between the ages of 4 and 8 years and may disappear at puberty. Sensitivity to flickering light starts around puberty. Some focal or partial epilepsies start in childhood and disappear after puberty. Complex-partial seizures may appear at any time since they are symptomatic. Tonic-clonic seizures may start at any age.

Although primary generalized epilepsy (idiopathic epilepsy) usually appears before puberty, it can appear later in life. However, epilepsy starting after puberty is more likely to be symptomatic.

22 Why do some people have their first fit in their teens?

Throughout early life right up to puberty the chemistry of the body is changing and developing. This means that some kinds of seizure will only be seen in the very young and will disappear as the child grows. Thus, many types of seizure will start in early childhood but disappear in the teens, whereas other types of seizure will start at puberty, particularly in girls.

23   Can people stop their own seizures?

People who get a long enough warning may be able to stop the attack by taking some action. For example, if jerking occurs in part of a limb, gripping that part firmly may stop the spread. If there is a sensation in part of the body a strong stimulus to that part may stop the attack. Some people can think and will themselves out of an attack.

24   Should I do anything to prevent my fit happening?

If you can learn some trick to control attacks, this may be a great advantage. Occasionally, stopping an attack by self-control can result in some brief emotional experience, e.g. a feeling of tension, or it may postpone the attack, which can be allowed to occur at home in safer or more acceptable circumstances.

25   Does epilepsy only happen in humans?

Epilepsy occurs in animals and birds and reptiles, though the type of seizure may not be the same as that seen in man.

Causes

26   What are the causes of epilepsy?

There are many causes of epilepsy and anyone may have a seizure under special circumstances if the insult to the brain is great enough. As will be mentioned in question 33, we all have an inborn tendency to have an epileptic attack and therefore in some people a low seizure threshold is the cause of their epilepsy. This is primary generalized epilepsy which used to be called idiopathic. In some people seizures occur because there has been some damage to the brain, either from injury or illness or disease. This is more likely to happen in those who have an inherited low seizure threshold. In some illnesses the chemical working of the body alters considerably and fits may then result. Some children are born with abnormal brains and because of this they have seizures. In a few people epileptic seizures occur because of a tumour in the brain.

27 Can epilepsy be caused by stress or a shock?

It is very very rare for epilepsy to be caused by stress or a shock, if by this we mean that the epilepsy started because of some stressful experience. However, it is common for seizures to be provoked by stress, anxiety or worry in those people with a low seizure threshold.

28 Can a bang on the head as a child cause epilepsy?

Nearly every child receives a bang on the head at some time. Although children are more likely than adults to develop epilepsy after a relatively mild head injury, it is unusual for epilepsy to result from a bang on the head unless the injury to the head has caused prolonged loss of consciousness and some other symptoms or signs, indicating bleeding inside the skull, or damage to part of the brain for example.

29 Can brain tumours be a cause of epilepsy?

Yes, but tumours of the brain are a relatively rare cause of epilepsy.

30 Can epilepsy occur with high blood pressure?

Epilepsy may occur if the blood pressure becomes raised or if there is damage to the brain caused as a result of high blood pressure, or a fit may occur because of hardening of the arteries of the brain.

31 An increasing number of young people take drugs nowadays. Do these cause seizures?

Seizures may occur if addictive drugs are used in high doses, or when such drugs are being withdrawn. Drugs used for the treatment of epilepsy are not addictive.

32 Do epileptic seizures result from whooping cough?

Epileptic seizures may occur occasionally in whooping cough, and occasionally from immunization against whooping cough. If the whooping cough is severe, part of the brain may be damaged because of lack of oxygen, and seizures may later occur because of this damage. In a predisposed child, any illness that causes a fever may result in a convulsion.

33 Is epilepsy inherited?

What is inherited is a tendency to have seizures. Evidence of this tendency is an abnormality in the EEG pattern called spike and wave. We know that this EEG pattern is inherited (though there may be no family history) and its presence means that the individual has a low seizure threshold, although they will not necessarily ever have a fit. A low seizure threshold means that the person is more liable to have a fit than someone with a high seizure threshold (see question 1). Sometimes epilepsy does appear to be more common in a particular family.

34 Will my children have epilepsy?

If one parent has epilepsy the chance of the children having epilepsy depends on the type and cause of the parents' epilepsy. Statistics on the inheritance of epilepsy are very complicated, and the values in the numerous reports vary greatly for various reasons. (See p. 2.)

This question can only be answered properly by considering the individual person. Statistics that do not refer to particular types of seizure but only mention unselected epilepsy, or seizure disorders, are not reliable; there are a great many of these. The figures that follow relate to seizures occurring in close relatives only. Close relatives are defined as parents, children or siblings of the person who has seizures.

It is important when studying the inheritance of epilepsy to separate out febrile convulsions. For example, in one study seizures occurred in 2.9% of the children of mothers with epilepsy compared to 1.7% of children of fathers with epilepsy. But if febrile convulsions were included, these figures were 11% and 6.9%. In one study of parents with tonic-clonic seizures, with or without an aura, 2.3% of the children had epilepsy; if febrile convulsions were included the figure rose to 9.2%. This study also compared tonic-clonic seizures without an aura (namely primary generalized epileptic seizures) and showed that 16.8% of children had seizures, compared to the 2.3% in the mixed group of tonic-clonic seizures.

Another large study showed that 5% of children of epileptic parents had seizures but seizures occurred in 3.6% of children whose parents did not have epilepsy. It is therefore very difficult to generalize, but it is possible that the likelihood of a parent with tonic-clonic seizures having a child with seizures is around 1 in 10, and a similar figure applies to parents with absences. Febrile convulsions are also likely to be found in 10% of close relatives, though the figures given by authors vary from 8 to 30% and in one study were as high as 50%.

If the parent has simple or partial complex seizures, the figure is lower than that found in primary generalized epilepsy. However, figures for the benign epilepsies of childhood are similar to those for primary generalized epilepsy.

It must be stressed that what is inherited is a tendency to have seizures and this is associated with an EEG pattern of spike and wave, and that this pattern may be found in the EEG traces of a number of close relatives, yet seizures may never occur. Finally, if the parents' epilepsy is a symptom of a known inherited disease the risk of the children having seizures depends on the genetics of that disease.

In general therefore there is no bar to having children in case they should have epilepsy, but detailed advice should be sought from a specialist in epilepsy, or a genetic counsellor.

35 Should I have my other child investigated?

It is worthwhile making an EEG on other members of the family to see if there is any spike and wave. If there is, it does not mean that they will have fits but it is a useful piece of information, especially if there is sensitivity to flickering light, because if one knows that a child is photosensitive one may prevent them having a fit whilst watching television.

36 My sister has idiopathic epilepsy. What risk is there to my children?

The risk of seizures is so slight (about 1%) that it can be ignored. Your children have a slightly higher risk of having an abnormal EEG, with spike and wave discharges, but this does not mean that they will have seizures (see questions 1 and 33).

37 Am I to blame for my child's fits?

It is quite common for parents to feel guilty about their child's epilepsy and to feel that they are in some way to blame. In Victorian times it was thought that the child suffered because of the parents wrong doing, but in epilepsy it is not true that the sin of the parent is visited on the child. Furthermore, the importance of a family history of epilepsy is often exaggerated, and no person with epilepsy should feel blame if their child develops seizures.

38 Is genetic counselling available for people with epilepsy?

Yes. If the epilepsy is primary generalized there is usually no bar to having children. If the epilepsy is symptomatic of some brain disease or disorder, the genetic risk depends on the particular disorder.

Genetic counselling is available in many centres, especially Departments of Child Health in teaching hospitals, etc. You should ask your family doctor to refer you for advice.

39 Is epilepsy an allergy?

Epilepsy is not an allergy.

Precipitants

40   How do fits start and stop?

Seizures may start because of chemical changes in the brain. In some people changes arise within the body and the precipitant of the seizure may be easily recognized, for example, hormonal changes during the menstrual cycle, or sudden change in blood sugar, or there may be emotional stress which causes internal chemical changes.

In some people seizures may be provoked by various sensory stimuli. These are known as reflex epilepsies and include seizures caused by sounds, music, reading, touch, hot water and flickering light. Such epilepsies are rare, apart from seizures provoked by flickering light.

Seizures stop when the brain cells are exhausted, which happens after quite a short time, usually only a matter of a minute or so.

41   Why do fits occur when they do?

We still do not know precisely why fits occur when they do. If only we knew this it would be easier to prevent seizures.

42   Can people bring on their own fits?

There are a number of ways whereby a seizure may be brought on. Some patients overbreathe, a few who are sensitive to flickering light may produce a seizure by rapidly blinking in bright sunlight, or waving their hand in front of their eyes whilst looking at the sun, or they may use the flicker of the television screen. In some patients an emotional upset will bring on a seizure.

43   Can stress or getting upset bring on an attack?

Yes. It is very very rare for stress or severe emotional disturbance to be the original cause of the epilepsy, but it is quite common for attacks to occur at times of stress, anxiety or worry. Some people may develop a pattern of having seizures under particularly stressful circumstances.

People whose attacks are clearly precipitated by stress can be helped, with professional guidance, to learn how to cope with situations that cause them anxiety or worry.

44   Do fits gets worse at times of exams?

Yes. In a few children, especially those who have absences with spike and wave in the EEG.

45   Does excitement bring on a fit?

It is quite common for children to have an increase in seizures when they are excited, but life would be very dull without excitement.

46   Are people more likely to have fits if they are inactive?

Yes. Seizures are uncommon when a person is active, and are more likely to occur when the person is relaxed, inactive, bored or drowsy.

47   Can fits increase because of over-eating?

No.

48   Will fits occur more readily by drinking water or alcohol?

Alcohol taken in moderation is unlikely to affect epilepsy except in rare cases. Regular daily consumption may affect the working of the liver and cause it to work faster and when this happens (induction of liver enzymes) the amount of epileptic drugs in the body may be reduced and therefore a higher dose may be needed. Alcohol slows you up — barbiturates and benzodiazepines slow you up — therefore if you are taking either of these drugs you may get intoxicated on a smaller amount of alcohol.

If you drink a large amount of fluid more quickly than your body can get rid of it, you may get water intoxication. Water intoxication means that your body contains too much fluid and when this happens (extremely rarely) you might get a seizure. Very occasionally this may happen if you are taking carbamazepine (Tegretol) so if you are on this drug you should not drink more than 2 or 3 pints of any fluid over a period of 4–5 hours.

49   Will hot climates be harmful for epilepsy?

A hot climate is not harmful. Very high body temperature in malaria may precipitate convulsions in children.

50   Will other illnesses make my epilepsy worse?

If serious illnesses disturb the working of the body, seizures may increase during the illness.

51   Does constipation cause an increase in fits?

There is no scientific evidence to prove that constipation increases fits, but it may happen in a few people. Constipation occasionally results as a side effect of carbamazepine (Tegretol).

52   Can a flashing light cause a fit?

Flashing or flickering light can cause fits, the most common sources being the television screen, discotheques and sunlight reflected from water. Fits only occur in people whose brains are sensitive to flashing lights. Photosentitivity can only be diagnosed from the EEG response to flashing light. Photosensitivity is found in about 1 in 4000 children. Although photosensitivity is inherited, the findings in an EEG of an abnormal response to flashing light does not necessarily mean that the child will have seizures.

53   Are fits caused by watching television?

People who are sensitive to flickering light may have a fit when watching television, particularly if they go up close to the screen in order to switch on or adjust the set. Even when the television is working normally, the screen flickers 25 to 50 times every second and most photosensitive patients are sensitive to these flash rates. In order to know whether a person is photosensitive, it is necessary for them to have an EEG whilst they are looking at a flashing light. With this test it is possible to find out whether anyone is sensitive to flickering light, and also to find out the rates of flicker which will cause an EEG abnormality and which therefore might cause a fit if the person was exposed to flicker for long enough. In the EEG laboratory exposure to the flashing light is only for a short period and this is quite safe and will not cause a seizure.

54 What sort of fits can be caused by flashing light?

The commonest fit caused by flashing or flickering light is a tonic-clonic seizure. Absences may occur, but focal or partial seizures are rare.

55 Are fits increased by going to the cinema?

It is very rare indeed for fits to be caused by flicker from films in the cinema, as the rate of flicker is too fast. Home movies are slower and have been known to induce fits.

56 Are fits precipitated by sitting in a car watching the scenery go by?

Yes. A passenger who can look to the side towards the sun shining through trees or railings bordering the road, will be directly exposed to flickering light. On the other hand, the driver, who has to look straight ahead and is therefore not directly looking at the flicker, will not have a seizure.

57 Is it safe to go to discotheques?

If the person is sensitive to flickering light there is an increased risk of seizures at some discotheques, depending on the rate of flashing and the colour of the light (white is worse than colours).

Flashing at a rate of five times every second, or slower, is safe.

58 Why do I have my attack on a Thursday morning?

It is uncommon for seizures to occur on a particular day, though some patients tend to have them at week-ends. The cause may be psychological, or due to increased relaxation or increased tiredness following lack of sleep. Only taking a careful history can answer this question. What happened on Wednesday night?

*59   I have fits only when I am asleep. Does this mean I shall
     never have them when I am awake?*

If seizures have occurred only during sleep over many years, it is likely, but not certain, that this pattern will continue and fits are unlikely to occur during waking. This is recognized in the regulations for granting a driving licence.

*60   Do people have seizures during sleep, and is this
     dangerous?*

It is quite common for seizures to occur during sleep. Febrile convulsions may occur in a sleeping child. In benign rolandic epilepsy, focal seizures involving the face and mouth may occur in children, during sleep. The child wakes and is usually conscious but cannot speak. These seizures stop, usually before the age of 15 years, and are not seen in adults.

Tonic-clonic seizures often occur during sleep. Seizures during sleep are not usually dangerous, and it is often safer and more convenient to have seizures in bed. A possible danger is suffocation if a soft pillow is used.

This problem can be overcome by the use of special pillows, whose design means that safety and comfort is increased. For details about these pillows see question 199.

61   Why do I only have fits after waking?

The most common sort of seizure to happen just after waking is a myoclonic jerk. Myoclonic jerks occur within the first half hour of waking. Sometimes a series of little jerks will end in a tonic-clonic seizure.

Psychological aspects

62   Is epilepsy a mental disease?

Epilepsy is not a mental disease. Seizures may occur as a symptom in people who have brain damage or disease and such people may have mental retardation or mental subnormality as symptoms of this brain damage or disease.

63   Are people with epilepsy mentally retarded?

People with primary generalized epilepsy are rarely mentally handicapped, though this may occur in those people whose epilepsy is a symptom of brain damage or disorder.

Most people with epilepsy have levels of intelligence similar to the general population. Those who have epilepsy and are also mentally handicapped require special care, and there is a growing demand from the staff of adult training centres, special schools and sheltered workshops for training sessions on how to deal with the problem of people who have this double disability.

64   Is there such a thing as the 'epileptic personality'?

The old idea of an 'epileptic personality' was based on observations of people who had lived in institutions for years and who had severe epilepsy and inadequate treatment. Such people were said to be self-centred, irritable, religiose, emotionally unstable and aggressive. They thought other people were against them and they were difficult to get on with, and they were also slow in thought and speech.

Some people whose epilepsy is due to brain disorder may be slow and have difficulty in thinking. Some people who are irritable, aggressive and awkward may have been like this even if they had never had epilepsy. On the other hand, it is not surprising if people who have suffered from the prejudices and ignorance of society and as a result have found difficulty in getting jobs or accommodation, or have been shunned by their contemporaries, or led a restricted life, regard society as being against them. They may find continuing difficulty in adjusting to life. In some people slowness and irritability may be a side effect of drugs.

Thus, the term 'epileptic personality' should no longer be used as it is not justified and reasons can usually be found, in each individual, to explain the symptoms or behaviour.

65   Will attacks affect behaviour?

Behaviour can be affected in many ways. Psychomotor seizures are a variety of complex partial seizures. Psychomotor means emotional and behavioural change as well as movement, in other words, an attack that consists of abnormal behaviour. In such attacks the person may carry out complicated actions without being aware of this. On the other hand, simple repetitive and pointless actions may occur, such as mouth movements, uttering sounds, grimacing, touching things, undoing buttons or clothing. The person is unaware of these actions, which are called automatisms. They may happen in absences as well as complex partial seizures.

Since the temporal lobe is the part of the brain that sorts out messages from other parts, and stores memory, abnormal brain activity in this area may result in very peculiar experiences, such as seeing or hearing things (hallucinations), and this may result in the person behaving in an unusual manner. Other peculiar behaviour in a seizure may result in the person going round in circles, or running away.

66   Are people with epilepsy aggressive?

People are aggressive for many reasons and those with epilepsy are no more aggressive than those who do not have epilepsy. During or after a seizure, when people are confused and do not fully appreciate what is going on, they struggle or even strike out if touched, or if their face is slapped in order to 'bring them round'. This is not aggression but is a natural defensive response.

67   Are people with epilepsy dangerous when they have a fit?

People are not usually dangerous, but they may push or struggle with anyone who interferes with them during or after a seizure. Occasionally, a person may throw something in a psychomotor attack, especially when hallucinating. In complex partial seizures behaviour can be very strange and onlookers may not realize that the person is having a seizure, so they may be thought to be dangerous.

68   Are epileptics violent?

The term 'violent' is often used by relatives to describe the movements and behaviour that occur in a severe tonic-clonic seizure, and they may say that it is impossible 'to control' the patient. Tonic-clonic movements of limbs are very strong, and no attempt should be made to control them because of the risk of dislocating joints or breaking limbs.

69   Are people with epilepsy more likely to commit crimes?

The relation between epilepsy and criminal behaviour is of longstanding interest. Recent reports have shown that serious crimes committed during or after epileptic seizures are very rare (in one study, only 2 out of 158 persons). On the other hand, many people with epilepsy are socially deprived and may tend to drift into crime, but their antisocial behaviour should not be regarded as due to their epilepsy.

Statistics

70   Is epilepsy on the increase?

Epilepsy is not on the increase. Because more people are prepared to reveal the fact that they have epilepsy there may be an apparent increase, especially in some countries. On the other hand, patients and relatives are often very frightened of epilepsy and will not tell anyone, even doctors or social workers. In some countries there is an increase in epilepsy due to head injury following car accidents. However, better obstetrics and ante-natal and post-natal care may reduce the amount of epilepsy due to damage to the baby around birth.

71   How many people in the United Kingdom have fits?

There are around 300 000 people with epilepsy in England and Wales, which works out at 8 per 1000 of the population.

There is no reason to suppose that the incidence is any different in Scotland and Northern Ireland. (However, see the comments on statistics, p. 2.)

72   How common is epilepsy in children?

A febrile convulsion may occur in 3 of every 100 children and in 60% of these there will never be another convulsion. Epilepsy is slightly more likely to occur in children than adults. Epilepsy occurs in 1 in every 200 adults, i.e. 5 in 1000. It is probable that it occurs in 8 in 1000 children.

73   Are men more likely to have epilepsy than women?

Epilepsy is more common in men than women. In some countries the difference is very marked, just because women come to hospital less often than men. Spike and wave discharges are more common in the EEG traces of women than of men and therefore seizures that are primary and generalized may be more common in women. This is certainly true of seizures associated with sensitivity to flickering light.

74   Are boys more likely to have epilepsy than girls?

Febrile convulsions, infantile spasms and Lennox-Gastaut Syndrome are all more common in boys. Absences, myoclonic jerks and photosensitivity tend to be more common in girls.

2

Diagnosis and Investigations

Information from the patient

75   What sort of questions will the doctor ask?

The diagnosis of a seizure or of epilepsy depends mainly on a
detailed description of exactly what occurred, including the
circumstances. Because the person with epilepsy may not be
aware of what happened, it is essential for the doctor to
obtain a description from someone who saw the attack. As a
seizure is due to the brain cells working abnormally, it may
be difficult for the patient to describe the unusual
experiences. The doctor will ask for a moment to moment
account of what happened from start to finish of the attack
and also what happened before and after the attack. Even if
the patient cannot remember what happened before or
during the attack, most people can describe how they felt
afterwards and such symptoms as a sore tongue or cheek,
wet clothing, severe headache and aching limbs are a helpful
guide.

Clinical examination may give the doctor information if he
sees the patient at the time of the seizure, but at later
consultations there is often nothing to find on clinical
examination. After a first seizure most patients will be
referred to a hospital specialist for further opinion,
investigation and possible treatment. The first seizure must
be investigated, though not necessarily treated. Since a most

important part of the investigation is the description of the attack, someone who has seen the attack should accompany the patient. The past history is important since it may throw some light on a possible cause of the seizure.

The doctor will ask about past illnesses, details of birth and infancy, the family and personal history, including menstruation. If there have been previous attacks, the doctor will want to know when the first attack occurred, how often attacks happen, what previous investigations have been done, and what previous treatment has been given.

76   Have I really got epilepsy?

It is very important to be sure that the diagnosis really is epilepsy and this is not always easy. It is probable that a fifth of the patients referred to special clinics for epilepsy, with a definite or probable diagnosis of epilepsy, do not have epilepsy.

The most common condition to be mistaken for a seizure is a severe faint. The diagnosis depends on careful and accurate history taking. In a severe faint (or syncopal or vaso-vagal attack) there may be twitching or jerking movements of the limbs and these may be mistaken for the clonic movements of a tonic-clonic seizure. It is quite common for persons who faint to pass their water and this may be thought to mean they have had a seizure. However, there is always some warning feeling before a faint, and usually some precipitant (standing in a hot atmosphere, or school assembly, or the sight of blood, or needles, or syringes for injections, or seeing or hearing about something unpleasant). After a faint the patient comes round quickly, is not muddled or confused and there is no headache (provided the head has not been hit in falling which can cause concussion). During a tonic-clonic seizure the pulse is rapid, during a faint it is slow or can not be felt at all.

Another cause of misdiagnosis is to mistake emotional or psychological symptoms (panic attacks, anxiety, outbursts of aggression etc.) for seizures. Epileptic attacks always tend to be the same, whereas psychological attacks often vary. Precipitants (other than flickering light) are uncommon in epilepsy, but common in attacks of psychological or emotional nature.

77 How can one tell the difference between a fit and a faint?

In faints there is always a warning, and the faint occurs in response to some precipitants (standing in hot atmospheres, the sight of blood or needles, or injections etc.). In fits there is often no warning and no precipitant and the onset is sudden. After a faint, recovery is rapid without confusion, sleep or headache, whereas all these are common after a tonic-clonic seizure. Jerking and incontinence (passing of urine) can occur in both fits and in faints and the EEG can be normal or abnormal in either.

78 Is it possible to fake an epileptic fit?

Yes. People who have epilepsy may fake a fit in order to gain attention or advantage. Faking implies that the person is consciously and knowingly pretending to have a seizure. On the other hand, patients may have attacks that are not true seizures but are sometimes called 'hysterical', and these are not 'faked' attacks but are due to psychological causes.

79 Are childhood tantrums fits?

Childhood tantrums are not fits. Instead of tantrums, some young children may hold their breath when frustrated or hurt. These are breath-holding attacks and are not seizures.

80 Is epilepsy like apoplexy?

The Oxford English Dictionary defines apoplexy as a malady of sudden onset which arrests the powers of sense and motion and may be preceded by giddiness, partial loss of muscular power etc. This description sounds like epilepsy, but the OED also says that apoplexy is usually caused by an effusion of blood or serum in the brain. Apoplexy, from the medical point of view, is a stroke or cardiovascular accident. The symptoms will last longer than those of a seizure.

81 How can I tell the difference between a fit and a stroke?

A stroke is due to the sudden stopping of the blood supply to part of the brain. It is more common later in life, though it can occur in young adults and rarely in children. It is usually due to changes in the blood vessels of the brain, causing them to narrow and finally to become blocked. It may be due to a clot of blood arriving from another part of the body and blocking a vessel in the brain. The symptoms depend on the area of the brain that has been affected, but usually there is some paralysis and disturbance of speech. Symptoms of a stroke last much longer than those of a focal or partial seizure, though occasionally (mainly in children) a short period of paralysis may follow a focal fit. (This is called Todd's paralysis.) If a stroke causes a loss of consciousness, this will usually be longer than that which occurs in a fit.

82 What are catalepsy and cataplexy?

These rare conditions are not epileptic. Cataplexy is a sudden loss of muscle tone leading to a fall, and may be caused by strong emotion, most commonly by laughter. Catalepsy describes a condition in which the limbs remain in any position in which they are placed, as if made from wax.

83 Is narcolepsy a form of epilepsy?

Narcolepsy is not a form of epilepsy. It consists of a sudden and overwhelming desire to sleep, sleep often being deep but brief, and although the circumstances may be conducive to drowsiness the attacks may occur in situations where sleep is not socially acceptable (e.g. when driving a car or during an important business meeting).

84 Is there any connection between epilepsy and migraine?

Epilepsy and migraine attacks are both episodic and may be genetically determined. There is some evidence that people with migraine are more likely to have epilepsy and that those with epilepsy are more likely to have migraine. An attack of migraine often lasts longer than a seizure and the aura in migraine is usually longer than in epilepsy. If migraine affects only part of the body (focal or hemiplegic) it may be confused with focal epilepsy.

It has recently been suggested that some migraine attacks in children or adolescents in which vision is wholly or

partially lost (hemianopic migraine) are forms of benign
occipital epilepsy. Very rarely an epileptic seizure may occur
in a very severe attack of migraine.

Electroencephalography

85   What is an EEG?

The EEG is a recording of the tiny electric signals produced
by the brain. It tells us about the activity of the brain at any
given time. It may show abnormal activity of the sort
commonly found in epilepsy and may indicate that part of the
brain is working abnormally. The EEG tells us mainly about
function, but not about structure. The computerized
tomography (CT) scan tells us about structure.

A number of small silver discs (or pads) are placed over
the scalp, and the recording of activity is made from a
number of areas. Depending on the EEG machine,
simultaneous recording will be made from 8 to 16 areas.
During the recording the subject will be asked to breathe
very deeply for some minutes, since this may increase or
reveal abnormalities, and to look at a flashing light, since a
number of people are sensitive to flickering light and this
may be a reason for their having had a seizure. Some
patients will have an EEG taken while they are asleep, and a
few may have a special recording using a small portable tape
recorder, which records the EEG for 24 hours or more whilst
normal activities continue. It is often necessary to have more
than one EEG test. Since an EEG recording takes only a
relatively short time, it is quite possible that there may be no
abnormality, so the test may need to be repeated.

86   Is it necessary to have an EEG?

An EEG is a simple and harmless test which gives
information about the working of the brain. This test should
be made initially in every patient who has a seizure because
it may help in diagnosis and treatment and it may be
important in future years to know what the EEG was like at
the start of epilepsy. It may be necessary to repeat the EEG
test from time to time.

87   Does the EEG give a clear diagnosis?

The EEG does not necessarily give a clear diagnosis; it may be normal in a person who has epileptic seizures and abnormal in someone who does not. The EEG does not diagnose epilepsy, although it may confirm the diagnosis. It may also help to decide the cause and aid decisions about treatment, e.g. whether drug treatment should be given or whether treatment can stop. Repeating the EEG after drug treatment has stopped may reveal the return of EEG abnormality, thus allowing the doctor to re-start treatment before an actual seizure occurs.

88   Does it hurt to have an EEG?

An EEG is painless but may cause slight discomfort. Electrodes, which are usually small silver discs, are attached to the scalp using sticky tape or glue, or sometimes pads are used and these are held in place by rubber bands. Salty jelly is applied between the electrode and the scalp, and slight scratching of the scalp may be made to make sure there is a good contact. If glue is used, it is removed with acetone, and combing the hair may be slightly uncomfortable if any glue remains in it.

89   Why is the EEG made while the person is tired or asleep?

In some sorts of seizure, abnormalities in the EEG are more likely to be seen during sleep or just after waking.

90   Should tablets be stopped before the EEG?

Tablets should not be stopped before the EEG, unless the patient is already in hospital and there is some special reason for stopping medication. Since most anticonvulsants remain in the body for many hours, or several days, stopping drugs for 24 or 48 hours does not help. However, all benzodiazepines can make the EEG normal so, if generalized epilepsy is suspected, these drugs should be stopped for at least 2 weeks before the EEG.

91   Will the EEG show for sure that there is brain damage?

No. The EEG may be quite normal even when there is brain damage. Dead brain cells do not produce electrical activity.

92   If my EEG is abnormal does it mean that I have epilepsy?

An abnormal EEG does not mean epilepsy. Relatives of a person who has primary generalized epilepsy may often show some slight EEG abnormality (spike and wave) without having any seizures.

93   If my EEG is normal can I still have epilepsy?

Yes. A single EEG is often normal in someone who has epilepsy. It may be necessary to make several EEG traces during waking and sleeping. Also, long recordings may be needed in order to reveal an abnormality. If seizures occur at special times (e.g. just before menstruation) it may be helpful to take the EEG at that time.

Other tests

94   What tests will I have?

The tests depend on the patient's history and the results of physical examination, and may vary according to the type of seizure and the possible cause. The most common tests are the EEG and CT scan, and some doctors will arrange a skull X-ray. Various blood tests may be made before treatment with drugs is started.

If the specialist has discovered some abnormality on physical examination, other special tests will be made since a seizure can be a symptom of very many disorders and diseases, not only of those involving the brain. The hospital doctor may carry out special tests to see if the cause can be found.

95 *Will a skull X-ray reveal the cause of epilepsy?*

A skull X-ray will only rarely reveal the cause of the epilepsy because it is not possible to see the brain on a straight X-ray. One may, of course, see fractures of the skull.

Before the invention of the CT scan, it was necessary either to introduce air into the spaces round the brain (this was a pneumoencephalogram) or to inject a special fluid into the arteries supplying the brain (this was an angiogram). With these two techniques the X-ray pictures gave information about the structure of the brain.

96 *Should I have a brain scan?*

A brain scan may be helpful in revealing the cause of the epilepsy, but it is a test that is not necessary in all subjects and the decision must be made by the specialist.

97 *Will a CT scan reveal the cause of epilepsy?*

CT or CAT stands for computerized (axial) tomography. A CT scan, which is a specialized X-ray, tells the doctor about the structure of the brain, and it may therefore reveal the cause of epilepsy. However, it may be normal even when the EEG shows a focal abnormality.

3

Treatment and Outlook

Methods of treatment

The first seizure needs investigation because there may be a cause which can itself be treated. Once the diagnosis of epilepsy has been made the appropriate treatment can be started. There are six methods of treatment, some being used very rarely. Most patients will be treated with antiepileptic drugs.

1 Treating the cause.
2 Avoiding precipitants of seizures.
3 Antiepileptic drugs (anticonvulsants).
4 Behaviour modification.
5 Surgery.
6 Diet.

Drugs

98   How many antiepileptic drugs are there?

There are more than 20 antiepileptic drugs representing 10 main groups. However, many of these drugs are rarely used, only eight being in common use as shown in Table 1.

Table 1   Antiepileptic drugs in common use

Generic name	Trade name	Preparations
Carbamazepine	Tegretol	Tablets 100mg, 200mg, 400mg Syrup 100mg/5ml
Clonazepam	Rivotril	Tablets 0.5mg, 2mg Ampoules for injection 1mg/1ml
Diazepam	Valium Stelosid	Ampoules for injection 5mg/ml Rectal applicator 5mg, 10mg
Ethosuximide	Zarontin	Capsule 250mg, syrup 250mg/5ml
	Emeside	Capsule 250mg, syrup 250mg/5ml
Phenobarbitone	Luminal	Tablets 15mg, 30mg, 60mg
Phenytoin	Epanutin	Capsule 25mg, 50mg, 100mg Suspension 30mg/5ml Tablets 50mg, 100mg Chewable (Infatabs) 50mg
Primidone	Mysoline	Tablets 250mg
Sodium valproate	Epilim	Tablets 100mg (crushable) Syrup 200mg/5ml Liquid 200mg/5ml (sugar free) Tablets 200mg, 500mg (enteric coated)

99   Why do some drugs have two or more names?

Drugs have a proprietary or trade name, usually given by the manufacturer who introduced the drug, and they have a proper chemical (generic) name. Thus, Tegretol is a proprietary name and the generic name is carbamazepine. Phenytoin is a generic name and the drug is also known as diphenylhydantoinate and with these names the drug can be made by any manufacturer. The trade name in the United Kingdom is Epanutin and in the United States is Dilantin, and drugs with these two names are made by a particular pharmaceutical firm.

100 How do antiepileptic drugs work?

Seizures occur when brain cells act or pass messages when they should not do so, and this results either in other cells being switched on (activated) or not switched off (inhibited). Some antiepileptic drugs make cells less excitable, others make it less likely for messages to be passed from one cell to another. Some drugs may increase the amount of a naturally occurring chemical in the brain which inhibits (stops) discharges. However, there is still a great deal to be learnt about how drugs work.

101 Is Valium useful in epilepsy?

Valium (diazepam) is very useful for controlling febrile convulsions and status epilepticus if it is given into a vein or into the rectum (back passage). It should not be given into a muscle because it will not be absorbed quickly into the body. There are special tubes obtainable from the doctor which make it very easy for a parent to give the diazepam into the rectum.

Diazepam is also used occasionally to treat anxiety in a person with epilepsy, especially if the anxiety or stress is likely to precipitate seizures.

102 How does the doctor decide the dose of drugs?

The prescribing of most antiepileptic drugs is based on the patient's weight, giving so many milligrams for each kilogram of body weight. Slightly different calculations may be made for children. Changes in dose depend on whether seizures are controlled or whether side effects (unwanted effects) occur. Measurement of the amount of drug in the blood (serum levels) tells the doctor whether the patient is receiving enough or too much of the drug. Patients differ in the way they absorb drugs and the way that they metabolize (change) these drugs in the body and get rid of them. For each drug there is an 'optimum' therapeutic range. If the serum level is below this range and the patient is taking all the tablets as prescribed yet is still having seizures, the dose may need to be increased. If the serum level is above this range the patient may have or may develop side effects.

However, the amount of phenytoin (Epanutin) cannot be judged accurately from the patient's weight and the increase and correct dose depend on the serum levels, so with this drug it is essential to monitor treatment with blood tests.

If a patient is not having seizures it does not matter if they have a low serum level of the drug.

103   Why do doctors want to change my child's pills if he has a fit and is taken to casualty?

The aim of treatment in most cases is to stop all seizures. If a child continues to have seizures, we have to decide why this happens, whether the daily dose is sufficient, whether the right amount of the drug is available in the body to control the fits, or whether we are using the right drug. The doctor in casualty may give an extra amount of drug to cover the immediate emergency, or refer the child back to the family doctor or to the consultant. Doctors only know if the drug and dose are effective if fits stop, and the re-appearance of any seizure means that further enquiry is needed.

104   Why did the previous doctor prescribe all these drugs, when you say some of them can be stopped?

For many years it was fashionable to use several drugs, in the belief that one could use a smaller dose of each drug and thus avoid unwanted side effects. In recent years we have learnt a great deal more about drugs and have been able to measure the amount in the blood. We have realized that one drug may affect another drug if they are combined and thus the addition of a second drug may lead to a reduction of or an increase in the effect of the first drug. A number of antiepileptic drugs make the liver work faster and when this happens the effective dose of any other drug is reduced. Drugs that may have this effect are phenytoin, phenobarbitone and carbamazepine, but not sodium valproate, ethosuximide and benzodiazepines. However, drugs may affect each other in various ways quite apart from the effect on the liver. Drug interaction is very complicated and this is a good reason for using only one drug. It always takes quite a long time for any change in ideas in medicine to reach every doctor.

105   What is monotherapy?

Monotherapy means treatment with a single drug. Polytherapy or polypharmacy is the opposite, and means using several drugs.

106   Do people who have seizures need to be treated with more than one drug?

If treatment starts early after the onset of the epilepsy, most peoples seizures can be controlled by a single drug. If the first drug does not work, another drug can be used and the first drug slowly stopped. If the seizures have been present for many years, and if the patient is already taking two or three drugs, it is more difficult to control fits with a single drug but it is still possible. Primary generalized epilepsy responds better to monotherapy than partial epilepsy because partial epilepsy is usually symptomatic of some brain damage, disease or disorder. Some of the severe childhood epilepsies are very difficult to treat and more than one drug may be needed.

107   Why do I need to be seen regularly at hospital?

Regular attendance at hospital is necessary to make sure that you remain free from seizures and are getting the right amount of drugs and that your drugs are not producing any side effects. Regular attendance will also give you the opportunity of discussing any problems.

108   How often should I see my doctor while I am on drug treatment?

At the start of treatment it is usual for patients to be seen every 2 to 4 weeks. Once seizures are controlled, visits are every 3 months and then every 6 months. The frequency of visits will depend on the type of seizure, the age of the patient and the drug used.

109   How often should drug therapy be revised?

If seizures are controlled and there are no side effects there is no need to revise therapy. This does of course assume that the patient has been told by the doctor what side effects might possibly occur with the particular drug being used. If there have been no seizures whatsoever for at least 2 years, it may be possible to revise therapy and possibly reduce the total daily dose of antiepileptic drug.

110   Do increases in drug doses ever bring on attacks?

Occasionally too large a dose of antiepileptic drugs may cause an increase in the number of seizures.

111   I have taken phenobarbitone for 20 years. Should I change to a more modern drug?

If seizures are completely controlled and if there are no side effects whatsoever, there is no point in changing medication. However, many patients who have taken phenobarbitone for many years feel much better in themselves when they are no longer taking this drug. Phenobarbitone and primidone, both being barbiturates, have to be withdrawn extremely slowly because of the risk of fits occurring during or after their withdrawal. No patient should therefore reduce or stop barbiturates without seeking medical advice.

112   Why should I take drugs if I still have fits?

If seizures continue despite taking drugs, it is possible that the dose of drug is too small or the wrong sort of drug is being used. On the other hand, fits might be even more severe and occur more often if no drugs were taken.

113   Should I have a blood test every time I visit the clinic?

Blood tests in epilepsy clinics may be done to measure the amount of antiepileptic drug in the blood, or to check that there are no unwanted effects from the drugs and that the body is working correctly. However, such tests should not be undertaken routinely, but only if there is some clinical indication.

114 When is it necessary to have blood levels of my drugs measured?

Measurement of blood (serum) levels of drugs are usually only necessary if the result of treatment is not that which is to be expected — namely, failure to stop seizures despite a reasonable dose of drug based on body weight, or the presence of possible unwanted side effects (e.g. drowsiness). If the patient is receiving several drugs and develops some side effects, measurement of the serum levels may reveal which drug is to blame. Decisions about increasing or decreasing the dose of phenytoin (Epanutin or Dilantin) depend on measurement of drug levels, because with this drug one cannot decide the dose on body weight with any accuracy, and very small increases in dose may result in toxic unwanted effects.

115 Can general practitioners measure blood levels?

General practitioners can take blood for serum levels, but the sample has to be sent to a hospital laboratory for examination. Interpretation of the results of tests depends on experience, and the so-called 'optimum' levels are only a guide. For example, a low serum level does not matter if all seizures are controlled on the present dose of drugs.

116 Must I take my tablets regularly?

Seizures are due to abnormal messages in the brain. These messages are passed by chemical changes in the brain cells. Drugs are chemicals that prevent unwanted or abnormal messages being passed. Therefore they must be taken regularly, every day, to control seizures.

117 Will I come to harm if I forget to take my tablets?

This depends on the sort of tablet. The body gets rid of some drugs quickly, whereas others stay in the body for a day or more. Missing only one dose or even one day probably does not matter, but if tablets are not taken for several days there is a risk of a seizure, and even of status epilepticus.

118   If I miss a dose will it be all right if I take a double dose next time?

Missing one dose does not usually matter, but you should not take a double dose next time.

119   If I take a larger dose of drugs will this work better?

You should never take more drugs than a doctor suggests. With most drugs the dose depends on your body weight. It may be necessary to measure the amount of drugs in your blood, especially to make sure you are not taking too much. Taking too large a dose can produce unwanted side effects, whereas too little may not control seizures.

120   What do I do about my tablets if I have a late night out?

Take the tablets when you get home. Most antiepileptic drugs can be taken once or twice daily. A few patients may have to take tablets three times a day. Although tablets should be taken every day at regular intervals, it does not matter if the interval is different on one particular day.

121   Should I always carry my tablets with me?

There is no need to carry your tablets with you, but it is wise to carry a card stating what drugs you take.

122   Is it possible to take all the drugs together?

If you are on several different drugs (including those for conditions other than epilepsy) you can take all tablets together at the same time, once, twice or three times a day.

123   How often should I take my drugs?

All antiepileptic drugs must be taken regularly every day. Many can be taken once a day, usually before going to bed at night. Most tablets can be taken twice a day, in the morning and in the evening and only in rare cases is it necessary to take tablets three times a day. If this has to be done the tablets should be taken first thing in the morning, in the late afternoon after returning from school or work, and the last tablet before going to bed at night. The interval between each dose depends on the speed at which the drug is absorbed into the body and the rate at which the body gets rid of the drug.

When we take any drug it is gradually absorbed into the body from the stomach or gut. After some time, usually a few hours, it will have reached its greatest level in the body, which is called the peak level. From then on the amount of drug in the body will gradually decrease, until the body has finally got rid of it all. The length of time taken for the peak amount to be reduced to half is called the half-life, and this is usually several hours. At this time a second dose of the drug should be taken to make sure that the level of the drug in the body remains high enough to control the seizures. The doctor decides, on the basis of the half-life, how often the particular drug needs to be taken. For example, if a drug has a half-life of 12 hours it can be taken twice a day. If the half-life is 20 hours or more it can be taken once a day.

124 Does it make any difference if tablets are taken before or after a meal?

If tablets are taken with or after a meal they may be absorbed into the body more slowly than if they are taken on an empty stomach. On the other hand, stomach (gastric) symptoms are less likely if the stomach already contains food or a milky drink.

125 If I have to be treated for some other illness, should I stop or continue my tablets?

In general, antiepileptic drugs must be continued during the time that other drugs are given for any illness. Because of drug interactions, change in dosage may be needed in some cases, and this the doctor will decide.

126 Will my tablets react with other drugs?

Many drugs have an effect on or interact with other drugs. Some antiepileptic drugs such as phenobarbitone, primidone, phenytoin and carbamazepine make the liver work faster and when this happens the body gets rid of other drugs more quickly, so the dose of these other drugs may have to be a little higher if they are to be effective. It is for this reason that a higher dose contraceptive pill may be needed. A few drugs decrease the ability of the body to get rid of other drugs. It is most important to check with your doctor.

127 What is a placebo?

A placebo is a substance that has no active effect on the patient. It may be a tablet or capsule containing inactive powder (sugar), or a bottle of medicine containing water and perhaps some colouring. The tablet may look exactly like an active drug. Placebos may be used in drug trials, so that the researcher can find out if the active drug is really effective, or if reported side effects are due to the drug.

128 What is the placebo effect?

Improvement may occur just because the patient sees a doctor and placebo effects are changes noted by the patient who thinks he is receiving an active drug, but these changes are psychological. The patient may expect the drug to make him better or if he thinks the drug will make him worse he may report side effects.

129 Is it wise and is it safe to have vaccinations or protective inoculations when one is taking antiepileptic drugs?

The fact of being on drugs is not important. The safety and wisdom of being vaccinated or inoculated depends on what disease is to be prevented, the age of the person, the particular risk to which they are exposed, and whether they have previously been vaccinated. A leaflet (SA35) called 'Protect your health abroad' is available from the DHSS and this gives advice relating to various countries.

130 Do antiepileptic drugs cause addiction?

Antiepileptic drugs given in proper dosage as advised by doctors do not cause addiction. A few of the drugs used in epilepsy may be misused, but they cannot cause true addiction.

131 Do you get seizures with addictive drugs?

Seizures may occur in association with an overdose of addictive drugs, such as heroin or morphine, or when these drugs are withdrawn.

Side effects

132 Do drugs have side effects?

Any drug that is effective can produce unwanted effects, or side effects. This includes herbal medicines. Sometimes the effects are due to taking too large a dose of the drug. These are 'dose-related' side effects. Other side effects occur because the individual is sensitive to the drug and these are called hypersensitive or idiosyncratic side effects and occur with a normal or small dose of the drug. There is no way of telling before hand whether someone is sensitive to a drug, and one has to wait until symptoms occur.

133 What are the side effects of antiepileptic drugs?

Many drugs produce similar side effects, such as drowsiness, giddiness, stomach upset. If a person is sensitive to a drug, the most common symptom is a skin rash. The side effects for each drug are well known and the patient should be warned about them.

134 Are anticonvulsants harmful?

Anticonvulsants are not harmful if used in proper doses, and if people are aware of possible side effects. If side effects are suspected from the symptoms, blood tests can be done to confirm this.

135 What are the long-term effects of drugs?

Many side effects depend on dose, and these are usually obvious to doctor and patient. It is more difficult to be sure about long-term effects, especially with barbiturates and phenytoin. It is therefore important for the person with epilepsy to be seen regularly and to have special tests if the doctor thinks this necessary, even if seizures are not occurring.

136   What can be done about adverse affects?

Patients should be told about possible adverse affects, and blood tests will show whether the drugs are to blame. Many of the adverse effects can be corrected by appropriate medical treatment but it is very important to recognize side effects in good time.

137   Why do you use phenytoin when it has so many unpleasant side effects?

Phenytoin is a very effective drug if properly used, but it is essential to do repeated blood tests. The side effects are more of a problem in children and adolescents than in adults because of the unsightly results such as an overgrowth of the gums, an increase in acne, an increase in bodily hair and sometimes, with long use, there may be some coarsening of the features.

138   My child used to be lively and intelligent, but he is not the same since taking all these drugs. Can I stop giving them?

Children are particularly likely to show side effects from drugs. If behaviour has altered since drugs have been taken, it is most important to ask for medical advice. The drugs should not be stopped unless this is advised by a doctor. There are many drugs to choose from, and a change may be needed if side effects occur. On the other hand, loss of liveliness and less ability in school work may be due to the epilepsy, or to psychological factors and not to the drugs.

139   Will drugs affect behaviour?

Phenobarbitone and primidone frequently affect behaviour in children and other drugs may do so. Some antiepileptic drugs like carbamazepine and sodium valproate may improve behaviour. The response depends on the age, the individual and the particular drug. If drugs control seizures, behaviour may improve.

140 Will drugs affect memory or concentration?

Drugs may affect memory or concentration if the dose is too high. Some drugs are more likely than others to affect learning in children. In people with complex-partial seizures, memory and concentration are more likely to be affected if the epilepsy is not controlled, or because of damage to the temporal lobe, since this is the brain's main centre for memory.

141 Can drugs make me tired?

Many drugs cause tiredness if the dose is too high or if the person is very sensitive to the drug, but tiredness may not be due to the drugs.

142 Can drugs make me irritable or moody?

Some drugs, especially barbiturates, may cause irritability, depression, or moodiness, in children and in adults.

143 Can drugs make me put on weight?

Some drugs may cause an increase in weight, especially sodium valproate.

Other therapies

144 Is it possible to treat epilepsy surgically?

Surgical treatment can help a small number of patients. It may be possible to remove a scar or a small damaged area of the brain. A decision as to whether an operation can help depends on detailed and specialized investigation by the neurosurgeon.

Although surgery may result in improvement, complete control of seizures occurs in less than half the cases, probably because surgery is considered as a last resort. However, good results depend on the proper and careful selection of patients.

145   Can seizures be controlled by a special diet?

Some types of childhood seizures may be controlled by a special diet called the ketogenic diet. It depends on a very rich and expensive diet mainly containing fats and oils. The diet now in use contains substances known as medium-chain triglycerides (MCT). This diet is cheaper and more acceptable, but it requires great skill on the part of the dietician and great patience and perseverance by the parents. It is used when antiepileptic drugs have failed to control seizures in children.

146   Do vitamins help?

Most balanced Western diets contain enough vitamins. Occasionally, some side effects of anticonvulsant drugs may be less if extra vitamins are taken. Treatment with some antiepileptic drugs (especially phenytoin) may result in a reduction of certain vitamins (eg. folic acid) and this may cause problems and require treatment. However, an increase in vitamins should only be made on medical advice, since an overdose of vitamins can be harmful.

147   Can I do anything to prevent a fit happening?

A regular routine may help to reduce fits — very late nights, lack of sleep, taking too much alcohol, should all be avoided. Also, see the next question.

148   Are there any therapies apart from drugs and surgery?

In some cases it is possible to *treat the cause.* Seizures may be a symptom of a disease or infection of the brain which can be treated by appropriate drugs, or seizures may result from a number of generalized illnesses in which the working of the body (metabolism) is upset. For example, in newborn babies, convulsions may occur because there is too little calcium or too little sugar in the blood, and correcting this deficiency will stop the seizure. If kidneys do not work properly, the body may become poisoned and seizures may occur — treatment of a kidney disease and correction of the associated chemical disturbance will stop the seizures. In a few patients the cause of the epilepsy is a nonmalignant tumour or growth or cyst which can be removed by the surgeon, thereby curing the epilepsy.

It may be possible to *avoid the precipitants* of seizures. People with epilepsy should lead as normal a life as possible, but the frequency of seizures may be reduced in some people if simple precautions are taken to avoid situations or circumstances that are known to precipitate attacks in a particular individual. People who are sensitive to flickering light (photosensitive), especially those whose attacks are associated with viewing television, may avoid attacks by watching television in a well lit room and not going near the screen to switch on or adjust the set. Most photosensitive people are protected from the effects of flickering light if they cover one eye with the palm of the hand. The effect of flickering sunlight reflected from water can be reduced by wearing polarized spectacles. Thus, a number of photosensitive patients can lead a normal life free from seizures, without taking drugs, by taking simple precautions to avoid the precipitant.

Some people learn from experience that they are most likely to have attacks after heavy drinking of alcohol, especially if they are short of sleep. Such people can reduce the frequency of their seizures by altering their life style.

In some patients *psychological treatment*, which modifies behaviour, may also lead to reduction of seizures. If children or adults gain from having a seizure, there will be a tendency for seizures to continue. If they learn that there is no benefit from having seizures, the number of seizures may be reduced. Alterations in attitude can be achieved by psychological treatment.

149 Will homoeopathic treatment help?

Homoeopathic treatment may help those who believe in it.

150   I have cured my epilepsy by taking health foods and herbal cures. Why don't you prescribe these?

There is no scientific evidence that health foods or herbal cures cure epilepsy. Doctors prefer to prescribe proven medicines. If belief in any treatment is strong enough the treatment may be effective. On the other hand, many people diagnosed as having epilepsy do not actually have it and in such people attacks may stop without any treatment, or because of a placebo effect.

151   Does faith healing help?

Faith healing is for those who have faith. Reputable faith healers usually advise that the taking of antiepileptic drugs should continue.

152   Is acupuncture of value?

At present there is insufficient scientific evidence to show whether or not acupuncture is helpful in epilepsy, though some people report benefit.

153   Do people with epilepsy need plenty of fresh air?

Fresh air and a regular life style help most people, including those with epilepsy.

154   Can a herbalists treatment cure epilepsy?

Very many different herbs have been used in the past, but there is no scientific evidence that any of them are as effective as proper antiepileptic drugs, and some herbal remedies may interfere with these drugs and cause trouble. Reputable modern herbal books do not recommend herbal remedies for epilepsy.

155   Can hypnosis help?

Hypnosis can help some people who have epilepsy, but it should be done by a doctor, and only if advised by the doctor who is treating a patient with epilepsy.

156 What is ECT?

ECT stands for electroconvulsive therapy, and consists of producing a seizure by passing an electric current across the brain, or one side of the brain, in a patient who is anaesthetized. It is therapy used by psychiatrists, mainly for severe depression.

Prognosis (Outlook)

157 What are the chances of drugs controlling seizures?

Primary generalized epilepsy (tonic-clonic seizures, absences, myoclonic jerks) and the benign partial epilepsies of childhood are easy to control if treated early and at least 80% should become free from all seizures. If seizures are due to some damage or disease of the brain (symptomatic epilepsy), especially partial seizures and the severe myoclonic epilepsies of early childhood, control is much more difficult and only about half the patients may become free from fits.

158 Do I have to take drugs all my life?

This depends on the sort of seizure and when the seizures began. Some patients, especially those with complex-partial seizures (temporal lobe epilepsy) and all patients whose fits are due to some brain damage or disease, should expect to take antiepileptic drugs for the rest of their life, perhaps in a lower dosage as the years progress.

159 When can I stop taking drugs?

Successful withdrawal of drugs depends on the type of seizure and the past history of the illness. Slow withdrawal of drugs is most likely to be successful in patients with primary generalized epilepsy (absences, tonic-clonic seizures and myoclonic seizures), and the response will normally be better in children than adults. Success is more likely if there have been no seizures for 5 years, and the longer the period of freedom the better chance of successful withdrawal of drugs.

Published statistics on the chance of relapse on withdrawal of drugs are not very helpful because they often refer to epilepsy in general, without separating the results according to the type of seizures.

The important factors for success are:

1 Primary generalized seizures or benign partial seizures of childhood.
2 A short history of seizures.
3 Early treatment.
4 Few seizures before they are completely controlled by drugs.

Re-appearance of seizures is most likely during the first 3 months of drug withdrawal, and if the person is free from seizures after being off all drugs for 6 months recurrence is less likely. If seizures re-appear during or after withdrawal, restarting drugs will control them.

The EEG can be helpful as a guide, and increase or reappearance of EEG abnormality indicates the need for restarting drugs.

160 How long after my fits have stopped might I stop taking drugs?

Depending on the type of seizure, the age at which the epilepsy first started, and the age of the person, it may be possible to try reducing the drugs after there have been no fits for 2 years. With some seizure it is necessary to continue drugs throughout life. Drugs control seizures, but do not cure epilepsy, just as insulin controls but does not cure diabetes.

161 Do you ever grow out of fits?

Many seizures that start in infancy or childhood may disappear around puberty. This is the rule in the benign focal epilepsies of childhood and frequenty occurs in primary generalized epilepsy (tonic-clonic seizures, absences, myoclonic epilepsy of early childhood). Seizures that are a symptom of some brain damage, disease, or disorder are unlikely to disappear with age, and seizures that start around puberty are likely to persist into adult life.

162 *Some children have convulsions and have no more*
after an early age, whereas others tend to continue
with fits. Why is this?

Children who have convulsions at an early age (6 months to 3 years) may have convulsions with a fever. As their brain matures it will no longer respond in this way. At least 60% of children with febrile convulsions have only a single convulsion, and only about 4 in every 100 may eventually have epilepsy. Some children with severe forms of epilepsy starting early in life will continue to have fits, though the type of seizure may change.

If there has been some damage to the structure of the brain, this will not disappear as the child grows older, and thus the seizures will tend to continue and may be very difficult to treat.

163 *For how long will I have epilepsy?*

It is not possible to generalize and the answer depends on the type of epilepsy and the type of seizure and the age at which the epilepsy started. Primary generalized epilepsy (absences, myoclonic jerks, some tonic clonic seizures) which start in childhood *may* disappear around puberty. Benign focal epilepsies of childhood *will* disappear. Seizures that are the result of some brain damage tend to continue and need prolonged epileptic therapy. Epilepsy that has been effectively treated from the start is more likely to disappear or to be controlled on a lower dose of antiepileptic drugs as time goes on.

However, we do not know the natural history of many types of epilepsy, or of seizures, because most people are treated with antiepileptic drugs.

164 *Is there any truth in the belief that the body changes*
every 7 years, so I can look for improvement in
seizures at the ages of 7, 14 and 21 years?

This belief is mainly mythical. It is true that some seizures which start in infancy (up to the age of 5) will disappear in early childhood, and this might coincide with the age of 7 years. Other seizures which start in childhood may disappear at puberty, which used to be around 14 years. However, there appear to be no evidence for a change at 21 years. In brief, there is no scientific support for the magical figures.

165 *My child went for year without a fit. Why have they come back?*

We often do not know why people have fits when they do. If seizures occur after a long period of freedom it may be due to the dose of antiepileptic drug having become too low or to chemical changes in the body occurring as the child grows up.

166 *If I stop my tablets will the attacks start again?*

Never stop taking tablets unless a doctor advises this. Antiepileptic drugs control seizures, so there is a considerable risk of having fits again if you stop taking them.

167 *Can epilepsy be cured?*

Epilepsy can be controlled with drugs, but cannot usually be 'cured', if by this one means doing something once and for all. A relatively few people with epilepsy can be cured if the cause is treated either by surgery, or by treating the illness that causes the seizure.

168 *Why do some people with epilepsy remain stable, whereas others deteriorate?*

People with primary generalized epilepsy rarely deteriorate. Deterioration may occur because of some brain disease or disorder of which epilepsy is a symptom. Some patients who continue to have very frequent or very severe seizures may eventually deteriorate. Prolonged over-dosage with some antiepileptic drugs may lead to deterioration.

169 *Will my epilepsy get worse?*

This depends on the epilepsy and its cause, and in part on whether treatment is early and effective.

170   Are people with epilepsy short-lived?

People with primary generalized epilepsy are not short-lived. If the epilepsy is a symptom of some particular disease, the length of life may depend on the nature of the causal disease, and people with severe symptomatic epilepsy have shorter lives than the general population.

171   Can people die from epileptic fits?

Death may occasionally occur if someone has a series of tonic-clonic fits (status epilepticus) and is not treated early enough. Occasionally, people suffocate during seizures in bed if they have very soft pillows. Patients may drown in a seizure if it occurs in a bath or while swimming. Most seizures are too short to cause death.

4

Living with Epilepsy

Coping with emergencies

172   Is it possible to stop a fit once it has started?

It is not possible to stop a tonic-clonic seizure once it has started. However, in partial seizures it may be possible to stop or shorten the seizure, or stop the progression to a tonic-clonic seizure. For example, if jerking starts in the hand, clenching the hand or gripping it with the other hand or having it gripped by someone else may stop the discharge spreading in the brain and thus stop the attack.

In complex partial seizures it may be possible to stop the attack by thinking hard of something. For example, if a person experiences deja vu, and thinks or even says to himself 'I have never seen it before' he may be able to stop the discharges in the brain.

173   What should I do to help if I see someone having a major fit?

Remain calm, and keep others from acting in a panic. Make sure the person is not in danger from traffic, fires, sharp objects, or falling from a height. Let the fit run its course and observe the following rules:

1   Do not try to force anything between the teeth to stop the tongue being bitten — tongues heal, broken teeth do

not. Do not try to stop any body movements; wait until these movements stop and the first deep breath is taken.
2 Turn the person on to one side placing something soft under the head.
3 Carefully loosen any tight clothing around the neck.
4 Stay with the person until he comes round fully but do not restrain him or try to 'bring him round'.
5 Once he is conscious, wait until he speaks to you.
6 Do not give him anything to drink.
7 Write down a description of what occurred during the fit because this is important information for doctors.

Fits other than tonic-clonic seizures rarely need any help or attention from bystanders, except for understanding.

174 Is it necessary to send for an ambulance every time someone has a major fit?

No, except under one of the following circumstances:

1 If a person is still 'fitting' after 10 minutes.
2 If another fit occurs immediately after the first one.
3 If recovery after the fit is very slow.
4 If there are obvious bodily injuries.

Day-to-day management

175 Is it advisable for people with epilepsy to live alone?

It is difficult to give a general answer to this question because so many factors are involved.

If someone with epilepsy has no choice but to live alone, a telephone would be most advisable and a good neighbour would be an obvious advantage. Fires and radiators should always be guarded, and a shower should be used instead of a bath. Anyone with epilepsy who lives alone should make sure that the social services department is aware of this fact and should ask for regular visits from a social worker. The social services might also be prepared to help with the cost of providing a shower, telephone and other aids.

Local authority housing departments will, where possible, allocate ground floor accomodation to people with epilepsy who live alone, and for whom high-rise flats would be a risk. Requests for such accommodation would need to be supported by a note from the individual's general practitioner.

If it is considered inadvisable for people with epilepsy to live alone, a period in one of the centres for epilepsy is an alternative. Information about these centres and how to apply for admission are given elsewhere in this book.

A useful book for those living alone is 'The New Source Book for the Disabled' by Gloria Hall (Heinemann, London, 1983).

176 Should I eat regular meals?

It is wise to have regular meals, and to avoid long periods without food, since prolonged lack of food, especially carbohydrates, may lead to a low blood sugar, and occasionally this makes seizures more likely.

177 Should I avoid or eat certain foods?

Very rarely an individual with epilepsy may be sensitive to particular foods and may need to avoid them. This sensitivity and its possible relation to the epilepsy can only be established by proper medical investigation. Most people with epilepsy can eat most foods. Unlike migraine, which may occur with specific substances, there is little evidence that epileptic attacks can be precipitated or reduced by taking or avoiding particular food or drink.

178 Is it wise to diet if one has epilepsy?

There is usually no harm in dieting provided it is done sensibly, using calorie control. However, people with epilepsy should be supervised by a dietician. A high-fibre diet is not advisable as it may interfere with the absorption of antiepileptic drugs and thus lead to loss of control of seizures.

179   Do I need more sleep than other people?

A regular routine is helpful, but every person varies as to the amount of sleep they need, and this has nothing to do with having epilepsy.

180   Is lack of sleep harmful?

Lack of sleep is known to be important in precipitating seizures and it should be avoided.

181   I feel my normal self after a seizure. Is it all right for me to carry on normally straight away?

If you feel quite all right and are not muddled or confused you can carry on normally.

182   Can I do anything to protect myself from injury in a fit?

If you have a warning and know you are likely to lose consciousness, sit or lie down, well away from fires, radiators, open windows or tops of stairs.

In the home all fires and radiators should be guarded. Furniture should be well spaced out and there should be very few sharp hard objects. In the kitchen, dishes should be carried to the oven for filling as opposed to carrying a heavy hot container from the oven to the table. Pan guards should be used. In the bathroom a shower is preferable to a bath and the bathroom door should not be locked. Some people with severe epilepsy may need to wear protective head gear to lessen damage in a fall.

183   Will I be able to manage the baby if my fits continue?

It is possible to manage looking after a baby if fits still continue though it is preferable to wait until seizures are controlled before starting a family.

184   I have frequent fits and have a baby? How can I reduce the risk of accidents?

Check with your doctor to make sure that everything possible has been done to reduce the frequency of your seizures and be sure to take your tablets regularly. Avoid carrying the baby as much as possible, especially up and down stairs. Change nappies with your baby on the floor. Whenever possible only bath the baby when someone else is present and make sure that the bath is firmly set on the floor.

You can get an automatic locking device fitted to your pram or pushchair so that if you have a seizure and lose control of the pram, the wheels will lock immediately. Details of this device are available from the British Epilepsy Association.

If you have particular worries, get in touch with your health visitor or social worker so that you can talk about your problems.

185   Will telling off a child bring on a seizure?

Yes, in some children, but it is important to treat a child with epilepsy in the same way as you treat other children. Children have to learn how to behave, whether they have epilepsy or not. If children realize that they can gain from having a seizure, seizures are more likely to occur, and the child will adapt less well to life.

186   My child always has a fit if he is out late, what can I do?

Children must learn as soon as possible how to deal with their own epilepsy. Assuming that they are old enough and intelligent enough to understand, they must be given a full explanation of epilepsy as well as responsibility for their own treatment. Many people only learn by experience that late nights or loss of sleep may cause a seizure.

187   If my son drinks he has a fit. What can I do?

Whether people have epilepsy or not they have to learn how they respond to drinking alcohol and the consequences of getting drunk. It is in fact uncommon for anybody to have a seizure every time they drink alcohol. Discuss matters with your son and ask for your doctors help.

188   What can you do if someone will not take his pills?

Adolescents dislike taking pills because it makes them feel different, and they also often forget. Most antiepileptic drugs can be taken once daily, and this is easier to remember. For those who forget (children and adults) the use of a container that is divided into daily compartments may help. Such a container is called a Dosett. It has compartments for each day of the week and four sections for each compartment. It is available from: Penmell Limited, 20 Ivybank Park, Bath, Avon BA2 5NF.

189   What inoculations or vaccinations should my epileptic child have?

All children should be protected against diphtheria, tetanus and poliomyelitis. Vaccination against smallpox is no longer needed. Measles vaccination should not be given to a child who has had convulsions unless special precautions (simultaneous administration of diluted normal immuno-globulins) are taken.

Immunization against pertussis (whooping cough) *may not be advisable* if there is a family history of epilepsy or if a child is already slow in development or has any disease of the nervous system.

Immunization against pertussis *should not be given if*:

1   The baby has an illness at the time which is causing a raised temperature.
2   There were any cerebral (i.e. brain) problems during the first month of life.
3   There is already a history of seizures or convulsions.
4   There has been any adverse reaction to a previous dose.

Immunization against pertussis should be made at the age of 3 months. BCG vaccination may be needed in some newborn babies if someone in the household has tuberculosis, and in some older children, depending on their response to special tests around the age of 10–13 years.

If rubella vaccination is to be given to a young girl, it should be before the start of menstruation.

190   We always see a different doctor at the hospital. How can he help?

Many patients and parents complain that they see a different doctor at each hospital attendance. This is less likely to happen in special epilepsy clinics, but there are few of these. One of the reasons is that junior doctors have to gain experience in treating epilepsy, so they have to be given training and some responsibility. Unfortunately, doctors in training often change jobs every 6 months or year. One solution might be to devise a better system of recording medical notes, so that the past history of the patient can be seen at a glance. This would avoid unnecessary questioning and make it easier for any doctor to give useful advice.

If you are not happy about your treatment, you can ask to see a consultant.

191   My doctor does not seem to understand or take an interest in my case. What should I do?

Ask your family doctor to refer you to a hospital consultant who takes a special interest in epilepsy. This might be a neurologist, a general physician or a psychiatrist. Where children are concerned, there are paediatric neurologists, and many paediatricians also take a special interest. If there is a conflict between patient and doctor, it is sometimes possible to arrange a transfer to another general practitioner. Your NHS medical card explains the procedure, and the Local Family Practitioner Committee, or Community Health Council will give further details. An excellent guide is 'A Patient's Guide to the National Health Service' by Angelina Hessayon, published in 1983 by the Consumers Association in paperback at £3.95.

192   The doctors at my local hospital do not seem to know what to do. What should I do?

Not all hospital doctors are knowledgeable about epilepsy. If your hospital consultant cannot help you, you can ask for a second opinion and this will usually mean referral to a doctor in an epilepsy clinic, or to a neurologist or paediatrician with a declared knowledge of epilepsy, or to a special centre for epilepsy. Most consultants should not object to a patient seeing another consultant for an opinion. However, you must not expect to receive *treatment* for epilepsy from two consultants at the same time — responsibility for treatment can only be taken by one consultant.

193 How can I explain epilepsy to my child of 5?

It is very difficult to explain epilepsy in a simple but accurate way to a 5 year old, but there is an excellent little book written for this purpose by Dr Roy G Beran. It is called 'Learning about Epilepsy' and it has a lot of pictures. It is available from Medical Education Services Limited, 36/37 Pembroke Street, Oxford OX1 1BL.

Another very good book is 'What difference does it make Danny?' by Helen Young, published by Andre Deutsch, 105 Great Russel Street, London WC1.

194 What will happen to my child when he leaves school?

A child with epilepsy has a minus in his/her life, and therefore that child must create a plus, the plus being something to offer in the way of qualifications when school days are over.

The school leaver with epilepsy faces employment problems, as do most young people. There is an excellent Schools Careers Service, and there are Specialist Careers Advisers. Before leaving school the boy or girl with epilepsy, and the parents, should make full use of these careers services.

Parents should be aware that children with disabilities have a legal right to remain at school until the age of 19 years, and local education authorities must provide for this eventuality.

195 What will happen to our epileptic or handicapped child when we die?

If both parents die before the child, and there are no relatives or close family friends to assume responsibility, the local authority would be responsible for the child's welfare until the child comes of age (i.e. 18 years), as would be the case with any other child. This means that the present medical and social care would continue.

Aids

196   Should I carry some sort of identity card?

It is helpful to carry a card stating that you have epilepsy and giving details about your tablets, and the name of your doctor or hospital. Such a card may stop people always sending for an ambulance when you have had a seizure and may even avoid your being regarded as 'drunk and disorderly' because of misinterpretation of your seizure.

'I have epilepsy' identity card is a small card (5½in × 4in) containing brief facts about the individual who carries it, along with simple first aid rules. The card is available free of charge from the British Epilepsy Association at the following addresses:

1   New Wokingham Road, Wokingham, Berkshire RG11 3AY.
2   313, Chapeltown Road, Leeds LS7 3JT.
3   Claremont Street Hospital, Belfast BT9 6AQ.
4   Guildhall Buildings, Navigation Street, Birmingham B2 4BT.

197   Should I carry an indentification necklet or bracelet?

Identification necklaces or bracelets have to be paid for, but contain more information and are therefore more helpful if you are taken into hospital and are unconscious. The following are available:

1   The S.O.S. Talisman, comes either as a pendant or a bracelet. The screwtop, heat- and water-resistant capsule contains a comprehensive information strip, on to which one should write all the vital personal details that may be needed if the person concerned is unable to give them verbally. There are sections for name and address, name and telephone number of next of kin and family doctor,

details of blood group, allergies, vaccinations, disabilities, in short anything that may be of help in an emergency. Each section heading is in six languages, so even when abroad the information can be easily understood.

The S.O.S. Talisman can be obtained from: S.O.S. Talisman Co. Ltd, 212–220 Regents Park Road, London N3 3HP.

2 The Medic-Alert bracelet or necklet is of stainless steel with medical insignia engraved on one side and on the reverse the appropriate medical warning, a serial number and the emergency telephone number. The Medic-Alert organization provides for any person with a hidden medical problem to have the protection of an emblem which gives an immediate 'flash warning' to hospital, doctors, police or other agencies who might attend such individuals when they are unable to speak for themselves, for example, during a seizure. Full information can be obtained from Medic-Alert Foundation, 11/13 Clifton Terrace, London N4 3JP.

198 Is it better to have a shower than a bath?

Yes, because drowning is a risk for anyone who has epilepsy, and a shower is safer. Taking a shower rather than a bath is particularly important for anyone who lives alone. Such people, if they only have a bath and cannot afford to install a shower, should contact their local DHSS and enquire about a grant.

199 Should one use special pillows at night?

Firm pillows should be used, but it is advisable to use a special antisuffocation pillow. This is made of porous foamed polyether, which allows air to pass through it and increases safety and comfort. The pillow can be washed by hand or washing machine, and should be rinsed thoroughly afterwards. Pillows are available from: Melco Products Ltd., Melco House, Market Street, Tottington, Bury BL8 3LL, Lancashire.

200   Is there any way of protecting the head in drop attacks?

Hospitals may provide special helmets to protect the head and these are made from shock-absorbent material covered with soft leather and secured by a strap. Some children may find that commercial helmets are more acceptable. For adolescents or adults commercial crash helmets can be used.

It is also possible to obtain a special helmet covered by a wig that is matched to the individual's hair colour and style.

201   How do I get a helmet to protect my child's head?

The helmet may be provided by the hospital. Helmets covered with a wig matched to an individual's hair colour and style can be obtained from: The David Lewis Centre, Warford, Alderley Edge, Cheshire SK9 7UD.

A 'venture helmet' has been developed for all adventurous children, to be worn whilst climbing, skating, cycling etc. Information can be obtained from: Innovcom Limited, South Bank, Daveylands, Wilmslow, Cheshire SK9 2AG.

Help from others — action groups, clubs, centres

202   Where can I get help locally from people who really understand the problems?

There are Action for Epilepsy Groups, run by the British Epilepsy Association, in many towns and cities in England, Wales and Northern Ireland. Members of these Action Groups all have experience of epilepsy in themselves or their families, and are often able to help and support those people who have problems because of epilepsy. Full details of the Action Groups are available from the British Epilepsy Association.

203   Where can I find out more about epilepsy?

From the following sources:

1   Your doctor.
2   Books such as those detailed elsewhere in this section.

3 Your local Action for Epilepsy Group, Epilepsy Club or Self-help Group.
4 The Epilepsy Associations.

In the United Kingdom The British Epilepsy Association can be contacted at the following addresses:

1 Crowthorne House, New Wokingham Road, Wokingham, Berkshire RG11 3AY.
2 313 Chapeltown Road, Leeds LS7 3JT, West Yorkshire.
3 Room 16, Claremont Street Hospital, Belfast BT9 6AQ, Northern Ireland.
4 1st Floor, Guildhall Buildings, Navigation Street, Birmingham B2 4BT.

Other organizations are:

The National Society for Epilepsy: Chalfont Centre, Chalfont St. Peter, Gerrards Cross, Buckinghamshire SL9 0RJ.
The Epilepsy Association of Scotland: 48 Govan Road, Glasgow G51 1JL.
The Mersey Region Epilepsy Association: 138 The Albany, Old Hall Street, Liverpool L3 9EY.
In the Republic of Ireland: The Irish Epilepsy Association, 249 Crumlin Road, Crumlin, Dublin 12.
See the Appendix for world-wide addresses.

204 Why isn't there more education about epilepsy?

This is mainly due to a lack of finance. The provision of education about epilepsy is the responsibility, for the most part, of the various epilepsy associations located in different countries. Films, videos and leaflets cost money to produce, and additional funds would be required for salaries of trained personnel. However, a great deal of educational work is maintained world wide, and is being expanded through the efforts of action groups. There is also increasing sponsorship of educational programmes by industry.

205 Are there any centres for adults with epilepsy?

There are currently seven centres in the United Kingdom for adults with epilepsy. Six of these are in England and one in Scotland. The adult centres provide long-term custodial care where necessary, but for most people an attempt is made to rehabilitate them after a temporary stay. Details of the centres in the United Kingdom are as follows:

1 Chalfont Centre for Epilepsy, Chalfont St Peter, Gerrards Cross, Buckinghamshire SL9 0RJ.
2 The David Lewis Centre for Epilepsy, Warford, Nr Alderley Edge, Cheshire SK9 7UD.
3 The Maghull Homes, Maghull, Nr Liverpool L31 8BR.
4 Quarriers Homes, Bridge of Weir, Renfrewshire, Scotland.
5 Cookridge Hall, Ridgeside, Cookridge, Leeds LS16 7NL.
6 The Meath Home for Epileptic Women and Girls, Godalming, Surrey.
7 St. Elizabeth's Home, South End, Much Hadham, Herts SG10 6EW.

Apart from these centres, there are two special NHS centres for adults with epilepsy.

1 Bootham Park Hospital, York Y03 7BY.
2 Chalfont Centre for Epilepsy, Chalfont St Peter, Gerrards Cross, Buckinghamshire SL9 0RJ.

There is one special centre for children with epilepsy at the Park Hospital for Children, Oxford OX3 7LQ.

A Handbook of International Epilepsy Centres was compiled in 1973 by the International Bureau for Epilepsy. A current handbook is being prepared by Epilepsy International, and further information is available from their United States Office at Las Palmas, C-160, 2855 Apalachee Parkway, Tallahassee, Florida 32301, USA.

206 How can we avoid being overprotective?

The simplest way to avoid being overprotective is to observe its effect on a child and to realize that it may be a help to the parent, but it is harmful to the child.

A child may need to be protected to a certain degree, depending on the nature of the seizure and its frequency. The sort of overprotection to avoid is the complete ban by parents of all activities that they cannot supervise, or which might possibly cause physical damage to the child if a seizure occurred. Such a ban prevents the child sharing in normal school activities, games and sports. The child is kept at home unnecessarily, and does not learn to be independent. The overprotected child is denied friendship and the pleasures of companionship and is made to feel different from other children. The consequent damage of this overprotection to emotional life is far greater than the possible physical damage resulting from having a seizure when not supervised or when indulging in normal activities such as climbing a tree.

There is an element of risk in allowing a child to lead a reasonably 'normal' life, but this is justifiable though it will often produce anxiety in the parent.

If a child's seizures are completely controlled, normal activities should not be restricted other than one-to-one supervision when swimming.

Restrictions

207   Can my child go out on his own?

The effect on the child with epilepsy who is not allowed to go out on his own is one that is too awful to contemplate, particularly as far as the teenager is concerned. Freedom to come and go is part of the growing-up process of all children, with or without epilepsy. The child who is prevented from enjoying his liberty and whose movements are always chaperoned, will find it doubly difficult to cope when schooldays are over, and he has to leave a sheltered home or school environment.

It is a good idea for a child with epilepsy going out on his own to have some form of identification, i.e. card, necklet or bracelet, so that assistance can be given if a fit occurs.

Young people who are photosensitive should be warned of the possible risk of going to discotheques and should also receive advice about drinking alcohol (see questions 187 and 220).

208   Can my handicapped child travel alone?

This depends on the age of the child, the nature of the seizures and their frequency and severity and the length of the journey. A short time travelling between home and school or in the local area may be perfectly possible, whereas a long journey somewhere abroad might well be inadvisable. The answer to this question must depend on the precise circumstances of the individual child.

209   Can my child do P.E. (physical education)?

The answer to this depends in part on the nature of the seizure, its duration and the degree of control of seizures. If children are no longer having seizures there is no reason why they should not take part in all forms of physical exercise, including climbing. To restrict climbing makes the child different from his peers and the risk of falling should be accepted by the parent and the school staff. Ultimately, the decision has to depend on the school staff who certainly should be informed about the child's epilepsy.

210   Can I play ball games?

Yes, except for water polo.

211   Can my child go on school-trips or to scout or guide camps etc?

The answer is yes, presupposing that the school staff are aware that the child has epilepsy, and in addition that they are prepared to cooperate. This latter is of special importance if the school trip is of several days duration because some oversight would be essential to ensure that the child took his or her tablets as prescribed.

Camping with a group can be a happy and successful experience for the child with epilepsy, but this does depend on those in charge of the camp being informed, and having a good relationship with the child and the parents. Those responsible for running the holiday should make sure that the child takes the medication, and that they know what to do if a seizure occurs.

Although additional supervision may sometimes be necessary, it is important that this be as unobtrusive as possible, so that the young camper with epilepsy does not appear to be singled out for special treatment.

212 Can I ride a bicycle?

Riding a bicycle on public roads in towns is quite dangerous for anybody of any age whether or not they have epilepsy. Cycling on private roads or parks or elsewhere is less likely to result in an accident to the rider or cause danger for others. Whether or not a person should be allowed to bicycle depends in part on the importance of cycling to that individual. It is obviously more dangerous for children to bicycle if they are still having attacks, but if all seizures have ceased, then the risk of cycling is probably no greater for someone with epilepsy than it is for someone without. It is probably wise for anybody who cycles to wear some form of head protection.

213 Is swimming allowed?

Everyone must learn to swim. No-one who has epilepsy should swim alone, whether or not their seizures are completely controlled. People with epilepsy who go swimming should be accompanied by another person who can swim well and life-save and who is aware that his or her companion has epilepsy. Supervision therefore should be on a one-to-one basis.

It is important to seek the doctors advice about swimming, and decisions will depend on the type of seizure, its frequency and whether there are known precipitants. For example, someone who is photosensitive may have an attack because of sunlight reflected from the surface of the water, and such people may be more at risk before they get into the water to swim than when they are actually in the water.

If swimming is part of the school curriculum, the teaching staff must know that the child has epilepsy. The school may not be prepared to accept responsibility, and it may be necessary for the child to go swimming either with a parent or with an older brother or sister.

Sometimes it helps in supervising the child whilst swimming in public baths for them to wear a very brightly coloured and distinctive swimming cap.

214   Can I go sub-aqua diving?

It would be unwise to take part in this particular activity, and it is unlikely that anyone with epilepsy would be knowingly accepted. Supervision of somebody swimming is relatively easy, but supervision in sub-aqua diving is difficult and the result of a seizure would be much more dangerous.

215   Can I go horse riding?

Yes it is perfectly reasonable for somebody with epilepsy to go horse riding as a hobby. You should of course always wear protective head gear. There is probably no greater risk of having a seizure and falling off a horse than there is falling off a horse without having a seizure. If seizures are not controlled, there might be some problems in competitive riding such as show jumping, and flat or hurdle racing would not be advisable because the occurence of a seizure could be dangerous to other people.

There are nationwide programmes offered by the organization, Riding for the Disabled, whose local address can be obtained from Avenue "R", National Agricultural Centre, Kenilworth, Warwickshire CV8 2LY.

216   Can I fly?

You may fly as a passenger, but bear in mind that long distance flights involve time changes and these affect the working of the body so you may have slight problems if you lose a lot of sleep.

There are restrictions about the granting of private and commercial licences. These are currently (1984) under review. Information should therefore be requested from the Civil Aviation Authority, 45–59 Kingsway, London WC2B 6TE.

217   Will I be allowed to foster a child?

If you have frequent major seizures then it is probable that the fostering authority will refuse the application. Otherwise, if the individual concerned satisfies the requirements that are demanded of any prospective foster parent, and the epilepsy is of no great consequence, then the fostering procedure should go ahead.

218   Am I allowed to adopt a child?

There is no reason in law why people with epilepsy should not adopt a child. In an 'informal' questionnaire survey carried out by the British Epilepsy Association in the 1970s, most adoption societies agreed that epilepsy would not constitute a ban. Today the local authority is responsible for monitoring the adoption process, and again, legally, there is no ban preventing applications from adults with epilepsy from being considered.

219   Is there any ban on people with epilepsy emigrating?

Emigration is becoming increasingly difficult for the general population, as more and more countries are prepared to accept skilled workers and professional people only. Those with epilepsy need therefore to have the same qualifications as their peers. It would appear that some countries do operate a ban on the entry of individuals with epilepsy, and it would be wise for any intending emigrant with epilepsy to check the regulations of the particular country. This can usually be done by contacting the appropriate embassy or legation, but it would also be wise to contact the Epilepsy Association of the country concerned.

220   Can I drink alcoholic drinks?

For many years doctors have advised people with epilepsy not to drink alcohol. In the days when most people were treated with phenobarbitone, this was perhaps understandable, because both alcohol and barbiturates slow up peoples reactions and they should not be combined. However, with modern antiepileptic drugs, recent research has shown that advice not to drink alcohol is not based on facts, and social drinking in moderation is acceptable. A few people (usually those with complex partial seizures) may have an explosive response to alcohol and they should not drink. (See also questions 48 and 187.)

221   Is beer safer than spirits?

Beer is not safer than spirits because the risk of a seizure after drinking a large amount of any fluid (beer, cider, water or fruit juice) in a short time may be greater than the risk of alcohol, though the risk is low with either. (See also question 48.)

222   Am I allowed to drive a car?

Yes if you have been free from epileptic attacks whilst awake for 2 years, or have had attacks only whilst asleep for at least 3 years before the date on which the licence is to have affect. It must also be shown that your driving is not likely to be a source of danger to the public.

223   I only have fits in the early morning. Can I drive?

It depends what is meant by 'early morning'. If 'early morning' means during sleep, and if fits have occurred only during sleep for at least 3 years, driving is permitted providing that the person has had no seizures whilst awake for 2 years. If by 'early morning' you mean whilst awake, you are not allowed to drive.

224   I always have a warning. Why can't I drive?

A warning is part of the seizure, and anyone who has seizures whilst awake is not allowed to drive. Warnings (or 'auras') may not provide sufficient time before loss of control or awareness occurs. In addition, people who have warnings may also have fits when consciousness is lost at the outset. Cases of especial difficulty are generally referred to the Hon. Medical Advisory Panel of the Department of Transport, where they receive very careful individual consideration.

225   Can I drive a dumper or fork-lift truck on a factory site?

Provided you are driving within the factory site, and have your employer's permission, you can drive a dumper or fork-lift truck because you are on private ground.

226   Am I allowed to drive a farm tractor?

You can drive a farm tractor without holding a driving licence if you only drive the tractor on the fields or private land and never go on to a public road.

227   Should I hand in my driving licence?

If anyone holding a driving licence has a fit for the first time, whether asleep or awake, driving must be stopped and investigation should take place in an attempt to find out the cause and assess the risk of another fit. If you have had a single seizure, you are not allowed to drive for 6 months or a year and you should hand in your driving licence to the driving authorities, and notify the Driving and Vehicle Licensing Centre in Swansea. If you remain free from seizures you can re-apply for a driving licence. If after your first seizure you take antiepileptic drugs you will be granted a licence for 1, 2 or 3 years but not a full licence. You only have to pay once for a driving licence, not each time you re-apply.

228   If I lose my licence can I get it back again?

Those people with epilepsy who have had their licences withdrawn may re-apply for a driving licence when they satisfy the amended regulations which came into force on the 21st April 1982.

The conditions are as follows:

1   Freedom from attacks whilst awake for 2 years.
2   Attacks have occurred only whilst asleep for 3 years.
3   Driving is not likely to be a source of danger to the public.

You write to the Licencing Authority who will send you a special green form on which you have to give details of the sort of attacks that you have had and the dates when they last occurred. On this form you will be asked to give permission for medical information to be given to the medical advisors by your own doctor and consultant who will confirm your own statement. Once this is done you will receive your licence again.

229 Am I allowed to drive a heavy goods vehicle (HGV) or a Public Service Vehicle (PSV)?

If you have had any seizure after the age of 5 years you will not be permitted to hold an HGV or a PSV licence.

230 Can I just drive in country lanes?

No, you cannot drive on any public roads.

231 How can I appeal against losing my driving licence?

It would be advisable for any licence holder wishing to appeal against a DVLC decision to discuss the matter in the first instance with a solicitor.

School and college education

232 Can my child go to a normal school?

Most children with epilepsy go to normal schools. Authorities have a clear duty to provide for children with special educational needs in ordinary schools. This means in effect that parents and young people seeking education in ordinary schools rather than in segregated special schools, do now have some legal backing.

The Education Act 1981 is the new law on children with special needs. A handbook explaining the meaning of the Act is available from: The Advisory Centre for Education, 18 Victoria Park Square, London E2 9PB.

233 Will my child's education be affected by epilepsy?

Absence seizures, which are brief lapses of awareness, may disrupt the child's concentration, particularly if they are repetitive and if the teacher is unaware of the situation. Such children might be labelled as inattentive 'day dreamers'. Early diagnosis and treatment are essential in order to minimize any adverse educational effect.

Major seizures will disrupt the child's performance temporarily, but if such seizures are infrequent or not too long lasting, the interference with the child's education will be minimal. The damage done will be considerably greater if the child is sent home each time he or she has a fit, particularly if the parent insists on keeping the child at home for long periods.

234 Should the school keep sending my child home after a seizure?

There is no need for this unless the seizure has been unusually severe. Teachers need to be informed about how to deal with a seizure in the classroom. Valuable learning time may be lost because of the interruption caused by the seizure itself, and if the child is then sent home further time is lost. Even more time may be lost because a child who is sent home on a Thursday is unlikely to return to school before the following Monday.

235 Will seizures be a bar to further education?

This is most unlikely, as all those institutions concerned with further education impose no ban on young people with epilepsy.

For those whose seizures are frequent and difficult to control, there are many colleges of further education which provide facilities for young people with all kinds of handicaps, including epilepsy. Details of these colleges are obtainable from your local education department or from any office of the British Epilepsy Association.

Children with epilepsy who attend Lingfield Hospital School in Surrey have provision for further education 'on site'. For further information write to the Head Teacher, Lingfield Hospital School, Lingfield, Surrey.

236   Should I tell the teachers that my child has epilepsy?

Parents should certainly inform the head teacher that the child has epilepsy. It may be that the seizures are well controlled, and that this particular child will have few if any attacks whilst in school. On the other hand, if a major fit (tonic-clonic) does occur, advance information on how to recognize and deal with the situation is most valuable. Another reason for making the head teacher aware that a pupil has epilepsy is that even if the seizures are only minor, they might impair the child's progress educationally. Also, some antiepileptic drugs affect learning.

237   Should the doctor tell the teacher the child has epilepsy?

Doctors only inform teachers about a child's health if the parent wishes this and gives written permission (this applies for children under the age of 16 — after the age of 16, decisions no longer rest with the parent, but with the child). Hospital doctors inform family doctors and also the school medical authorities and vice versa. The school medical authorities may inform the head teacher.

238   Should the teacher tell the doctor the child has fits?

Teachers may be the first to notice seizures such as absences, and it is certainly of help to a doctor to receive a description of a child's seizure from a teacher. Usually, teachers in the first instance inform parents, though they may tell the head teacher so that information can be given to the school medical authorities. Teachers often express concern to the parents over school performance, and tend to attribute slowness and poor performance to the effect of drugs. Such effects used to be common with phenobaritone and phenytoin, but they are uncommon with carbamazepine, sodium valproate and ethosuximide, drugs that are increasingly used for treatment of children in preference to the older drugs.

239   Are there special schools for the child with epilepsy?

In the United Kingdom there are five special schools for children with epilepsy:

Lingfield Hospital School,
Lingfield,
Surrey.
Tel: 0342 832243

There is a further education unit with the school to provide help for the handicapped school leavers.

Chilton School,
The Maghull Homes,
Deyes Lane,
Maghull,
Liverpool L31 6DJ.
Tel: 051 526 4133 Ext. 37

St Elizabeth's School,
South End,
Much Hadham,
Herts SG10 6EW.
Tel: 027 984 2233/4

Administered by the Order of the Daughters of the Cross

The David Lewis School,
The David Lewis Centre
   for Epilepsy,
Warford,
Alderley Edge,
Cheshire SK9 7UD.
Tel: 056 587 2153/2204

The school offers facilities for children who are academically able to remain to the age of 19 for further education at a local college.

Sedgwick House School,
Sedgwick,
Kendal,
Cumbria LA8 0YJ.
Tel: 0448 60352.

A recommendation to close this school has been made by the local authority, but is subject to confirmation by the Secretary of State. If the order is confirmed, then Sedgwick House will close in July 1985.

240   Who pays the fees for children in special schools?

The fees are paid by the Department of Education in the local authority from which the child comes.

241   Why were we not told earlier about Boarding Schools?

Possibly because it has become policy to emphasize the desirability of educating all children in ordinary schools unless the child's condition is so disabling that he or she cannot be integrated in this way. A clearer awareness of the child's special educational needs is essential so that if Residential School is the answer, placement can be made at an early age.

242   Will attacks affect learning?

Frequent absences may affect learning, but even quite short episodes of spike and wave (lasting less than 3 seconds) may affect learning. There is also evidence that learning may be affected in people with complex partial seizures if the EEG shows frequent very brief abnormalities, even though there is no apparent seizure.

243   Will drugs affect learning?

Overdosage with any drug may affect learning but learning in children may be affected by normal therapeutic doses of phenobarbitone, primidone or phenytoin. Benzodiazepines often slow up children and interfere with learning. Ethosuximide (Zarontin), sodium valproate (Epilim, Depakine) and carbamazepine (Tegretol) have the least effect on learning.

244   Will tablets affect my studies?

Barbiturates can affect studies in an adult just as they affect learning in a child. Benzodiazepines may also cause general slowing. Overdosage with other drugs may affect studying but this is easily corrected.

245   What information is available for teachers?

There are many leaflets available for teachers from the Epilepsy Associations. These leaflets deal with the problem of coping with a seizure in the classroom, types of seizures, medication, classroom first aid, school activities and careers.

There is information on swimming, camping and holidays.

The British Epilepsy Association provides a service of illustrated lectures and seminars for teachers, both those in ordinary schools and special schools.

In the case of student teachers, a similar service is offered as part of the curriculum in Colleges of Education and also to the staffs of Higher Education and Further Education establishments.

Employment

246   What kind of job can I do?

The suitability of the job depends on a number of factors such as the type of seizure, the frequency and severity, whether or not it occurs only during sleep and whether or not there is an adequate warning. If seizures are completely controlled people with epilepsy can do most jobs, provided that they have the right qualifications.

Since a licence to drive a heavy goods vehicle or public service vehicle will not be granted to anyone who has had seizures after the age of 5 years, these jobs are excluded.

247   Are there any jobs I should not do?

You cannot drive a heavy goods vehicle or public services vehicle if you have had any seizure after the age of 5. People with epilepsy, whether fully controlled or not, will not be acceptable in the Armed Forces. If you are entitled to hold a driving licence, you should be able to do most jobs, though one that involves always working at a considerable height would not be advisable.

248   What professions are closed to people with epilepsy?

None. However, successful entry into some professions may depend upon the length of the period during which the applicant with epilepsy has been seizure free, and may only be possible if the applicant's seizures are well controlled and health standards in general are satisfactory. People with epilepsy, who possess the right qualifications, are often more readily accepted into the profession of their choice than those individuals with epilepsy who seek employment of a non-professional nature.

Persistence and determination may well be needed, but successful entry can be expected.

249   Would I be allowed to work with children?

Unless the seizures are well controlled it is highly unlikely that a person with epilepsy would be allowed to train as a nursery nurse, and even with complete seizure control the employing authority may reject such a candidate because of the potential risk should a fit occur whilst the child is being handled. It should be less difficult for the individual who has epilepsy to obtain work with older children (see the section on teaching).

For those people with epilepsy whose seizures preclude them from working with small children, a 2 year course in community care or residential care might be the answer because the training would not only qualify them for the job, but also this 2 year period would perhaps see an improvement in seizure control.

Details of these and other courses can be obtained from colleges of higher education and colleges of further education.

250   Can I work near machinery?

The Health and Safety at Work Act 1974 says that employers must do 'what is reasonably practicable' to safeguard their employees' health and safety. This makes it essential for the employer to know which of his employees has epilepsy and is likely to have a seizure. Knowing this, the employer can then assess what the risks are and try to minimize them, particularly where moving machinery is involved. For some people with epilepsy it may therefore be perfectly safe to work near machinery, whereas for others the hazard is too great. It is not possible to generalize.

251   Would it be possible to train as a nurse?

The Department of Health and Social Security has not made any special recommendations on the employment of nurses with epilepsy. This confirms the fact that there are no regulations preventing the entry of people with epilepsy into the nursing profession. Schools of nursing vary in their reactions to applicants with epilepsy, and therefore the would-be nurse may need to 'shop around'.

It is extremely difficult for anyone with epilepsy to obtain pupil midwife training. A statement put out by the Central Midwives Board on 29 November 1979 made it clear that an applicant who has epilepsy may be considered who has been free from attacks *without* medication for a period of at least 2 years.

252 Can I become a teacher?

There are a number of subject areas where, because of the potential risks to pupils, continuous alertness is particularly important. These include physical education, home economics, chemistry and associated subjects. Candidates who suffer from conditions that may adversely affect such alertness (i.e. candidates with epilepsy), or any condition causing partial or complete loss of consciousness, should not generally be considered for training as teachers in these subjects.

For further information, application should be made to the Department of Education and Science, Elizabeth House, York Road, London SE1 7PH for a copy of Circular 11/78 'Medical Fitness of Teachers and of Entrants to Teacher Training'.

253 Can I enter the Armed Forces?

The Armed Forces will not accept anybody who has epilepsy on entry.

254 Do the police accept persons with epilepsy?

The police will not accept anyone with epilepsy on entry, but in some circumstances those who develop epilepsy may be retained in the police force.

255   Will the Merchant Navy accept people with epilepsy?

No. The Medical Standards for Seafarers — Merchant Shipping Notice No. M1061 — precludes all people with a history of epilepsy from seafaring.

The British Epilepsy Association has submitted comments to the Working Party to Review Medical Standards, stating that in its opinion the fact that epilepsy can be well controlled by anticonvulsant medication is not reflected in the Medical Standards, and therefore unnecessarily penalizes some people with epilepsy who could usefully perform some job at sea without jeopardizing their own safety or that of others.

256   Why can't I get a job because I have epilepsy?

People with epilepsy have difficulty in obtaining work largely because of prejudice and discrimination. Employers in general have little knowledge of epilepsy, and tend to assume that all seizures are major seizures, frightening, dramatic and time consuming with consequent disturbance to routine and even loss of production. Another reason for those with epilepsy finding it hard to get work is the attitude of other employees who may object to having such an individual working with them. It is very important for anyone with epilepsy to have qualifications that are at least equal to those of the other applicants for a particular post. Failure to get work may sometimes be blamed on the epilepsy when the real reason for being rejected is a lack of qualifications.

257   Are there any employment training schemes?

A course of work preparation and assessment at an employment rehabilitation centre may be suggested by the disablement resettlement officer (DRO). This may lead to training at a government skill centre, a specialist training college for disabled people, or a commercial college. For further information enquiries should be made at the local Jobcentre or employment office.

258   Should I register as a disabled person?

You should ask advice from the disablement resettlement officer who will be found at the local Jobcentre. These officers can also give information about courses of assessment at employment rehabilitation centres. What the DROs can offer to those who chose to register as disabled is not sympathy, but a realistic and positive approach in helping them achieve employment to match their abilities.

259   What is a disablement resettlement officer?

The disablement resettlement officer (DRO) exists within the framework of the employment service of the Manpower Services Commission and gives advice to intending employers of people with epilepsy. DROs are based at the local Jobcentre and have been specially selected and trained for the work of helping disabled people with a variety of handicaps to get and keep suitable jobs.

260   Are employers legally obliged to employ a number of handicapped people?

A scheme known as the Quota Scheme was established by the Disabled Persons (Employment) Act 1944 and provides that employers with 20 or more employees have a duty to employ at least 3% disabled people. For some time now there has been concern at the interpretation by some employers of the word 'duty', and it would seem that any attempt to enforce employers by legal means to comply with their 'duty' would be impractical.

   In July 1982, the Secretary of State for Employment announced that the Quota Scheme for the employment of disabled people was to be retained for the time being, but the Manpower Services Commission would be asked to draft a code of practice backed by a more general statutory duty.

261   Should I tell my employer that I have epileptic fits?

Yes. Many people with epilepsy do not disclose this fact when completing job applications or when being interviewed. Should seizures then occur whilst at work, the individual may be dismissed without recourse to an industrial tribunal.

262 *Do I have to declare epilepsy when applying for a job?*

There is nothing of which to be ashamed in having epilepsy, so, for the sake of self-esteem and self-respect, the job applicant with epilepsy should declare it. However, the choice is with the applicant, as declaration is not compulsory. Should the applicant conceal the fact of epilepsy and the matter comes to light at a later stage, the employer may feel that he has been deceived and dismiss the employee concerned. Having concealed the epilepsy, the sacked employee has little chance of successfully claiming for unfair dismissal.

From the point of view of safety at work, it is advisable for the job applicant with epilepsy to be open about it because the employer can then try to ensure that the risk of accidents is minimal. Sometimes an appropriate certificate from a general practitioner or consultant in support of a person's fitness for work may be of help.

263 *What should I tell an employer when I apply for a job?*

At the interview, make it clear what qualifications you have and the kind of job you want to do. Make sure the employer understands first and foremost that you can make a positive contribution to his business, because he is not employing people out of a sense of charity.

It is important for your employer to understand about your particular epilepsy. It is helpful to obtain a simple but factually written account from a doctor, which can either be presented to an employer or a personnel manager or to the doctor who may examine you before accepting you as medically fit for employment with the firm. Such a letter should describe the seizure, saying when you had the last one or, if they are still occurring, how often you have them. It should also state that you are on medication and that there are no side effects from your drugs. It is best if such a letter is addressed by name to the person concerned, rather than being headed 'To whom it may concern'.

*264   If I develop epilepsy after starting my job, should I tell
        my colleagues and my employer?*

It would be wise to inform your employer and your
colleagues because:

1   The employer is required by law to ensure safety at work
    for all his employees. He therefore must know of any
    change in an individual, so that he can re-assess the
    situation.
2   Colleagues need to be aware of what exactly happens if
    and when a fit occurs, and be able to help if necessary.

The employee who develops epilepsy should also inform
both employer and fellow workers because it will enable
them to see that their colleague newly diagnosed as having
epilepsy is no different in human terms from the person they
previously knew.

265   Should I do shift work?

Only if the shifts are of long duration. Those that change no
more often than every 2 to 3 months might be acceptable.
Shifts that change every 1 or 2 weeks should be avoided.
There should also be several days between each change of
shift. In general, shift work should be avoided if at all
possible.

*266   Would full-time work make me more likely to have
        fits?*

Epilepsy was once described as 'the enemy that attacks the
idle mind'. Generally speaking, the man or woman with
epilepsy who is gainfully and usefully occupied will have
fewer seizures than would otherwise be the case. It has
frequently been shown that those people with epilepsy in
full-time employment are as capable as their peers, and that
a normal days work is something with which people with
epilepsy can cope, with no adverse effects. Many people with
epilepsy have a better than average work record.

267 Am I covered by employer's insurance and are employers liable if I injure myself in a fit at work?

Insurance companies have undertaken, in general, to include *all* disabled people (and this includes people with epilepsy) in employers' liability insurance policies on the same terms as the able bodied. *Special insurance cover is not required*, but this is on the understanding that the employer, in allocating work, takes account of the nature of the disability, and he must therefore be aware that his employee has epilepsy.

268 Can employees with epilepsy be superannuated?

Yes. In June 1977, the Occupational Pensions Board reported on pension scheme cover for disabled people, including those with epilepsy. In their opinion, disabled people should have the same rights to pension schemes as the able bodied. Some superannuation schemes may present difficulties for people with epilepsy, and if so, advice should be sought from the British Epilepsy Association.

269 Was my employer right to sack me because of epilepsy?

If an employee has been open and honest with the employer about epilepsy, makes every attempt to keep good time at work and does his job to the satisfaction of the employer, then it is most certainly wrong for the employer to sack such an employee. However, there will always be a few individuals with epilepsy (as with other handicaps) who 'use' the epilepsy as an excuse for bad time keeping and shoddy work. In such cases, after giving the statutory warnings, the employer would certainly be justified in dismissing the employee concerned.

270 If I am sacked because of epilepsy, can I appeal or claim compensation?

Providing an employer was aware of the fact that an employee had epilepsy at the time that employee was appointed (and this underlines the need for an employee to inform the employer in the very first instance), then the employee has recourse to action if he or she is dismissed because of epilepsy.

Any employee contemplating a claim against an employer for unfair dismissal should first take advice from:

1 The appropriate trades union of which the employee is a member.
2 The Law Society.
3 The Citizens Advice Bureau.

Further advice on how to proceed can be obtained from any of the epilepsy associations, and more detailed information is available in a booklet entitled 'Your Rights at Work', which is Volume 2 in the 'Know Your Rights' series. This booklet is obtainable from the offices of the National Council for Civil Liberties, 186 King's Cross Road, London WC1X 9DE.

Sex and personal relationships

Menstruation

271 Why are my attacks usually before my periods and does menstruation affect the seizure pattern?

There is a change in the sex hormones before the start of the period, and this may cause a number of premenstrual symptoms. In some women there may be an increase in seizures at this time. However, some people, both male and female, tend to have their seizures at regular intervals. Thus, we are not sure whether seizures are really associated with the menstrual cycle and, if they are, we do not yet fully understand why. In order to decide if there may be a relation between seizures and the menstrual cycle it is necessary to keep a record of the seizures and the periods for at least 6 months.

Occasionally, seizures may increase at the time of ovulation. Changes in the EEG often occur at different times in the menstrual cycle.

272 Should I increase my drugs when I am due for a period?

It is not usually helpful to increase antiepileptic drugs when a period is due. If there is clear evidence that seizures always occur premenstrually, it may be possible to use hormonal treatment at this time.

273 Why should I take tablets all the time, when I only have fits during my period?

Some drugs act very quickly in a matter of hours, whereas others take several days. For this reason, it is necessary to take tablets regularly. Also, although seizures may seem to occur only around the time of a period, it is not always possible to be sure that this pattern will continue.

274 Would a hysterectomy help my epilepsy?

There is no scientific evidence that a hysterectomy (removal of the womb) will help epilepsy.

Marriage

275 Can I get married? Should I tell my fiancé(e) about my epilepsy?

You can certainly get married, but you must tell your fiancé(e) because you have to share your lives together.

276 Will I have normal married life?

Sexual desire is reduced in some people with epilepsy. It is always very difficult to know the reason for reduced sex drive, because there are many causes, amongst which psychological factors may be very important. Some patients with temporal lobe epilepsy may have a reduced sex drive.

277 Will sexual intercourse bring on a fit and is too much sex the cause of epilepsy?

It is very rare indeed for sexual intercourse to bring on a fit and there is no evidence that too much sex causes epilepsy.

278   Will my antiepileptic drugs affect my sex life?

Sometimes some of the antiepileptic drugs may affect sex hormones. Anyone who is worried about this should seek specialist advice.

Contraception

279   *Will the contraceptive pill interfere with my drugs for epilepsy?*

Contraceptive pills will not interfere with antiepileptic drugs.

289   *Can I use the pill for contraception?*

It is rare for the pill to cause an increase in seizures. It may well lead to improvement of the epilepsy, particularly if periods are irregular or if there is evidence that seizures are more likely to occur during the days before the start of a period.

281   *Do antiepileptic drugs interfere with the action of the pill?*

Some antiepileptic drugs (phenytoin, barbiturates, carbamazepine) may reduce the effect of the low-dose pill and thus cause an unwanted pregnancy. If you are already taking antiepileptic drugs before going on the pill, tell the doctor which drugs you are taking so he can prescribe the correct sort of pill.

Pregnancy

282   *Will epilepsy interfere with my having children?*

Not usually, but there is some evidence that people with epilepsy are slightly less likely to become pregnant. There is also some evidence that sex drive is reduced in some people with epilepsy and also that some drugs reduce sex drive.

However, fertility depends on very many factors, as does the sex drive, and this question can only be answered for each individual.

283 Is pregnancy dangerous for someone with epilepsy?

In about half the people with epilepsy who become pregnant there would be no change in their seizures, but a quarter may improve and in a quarter there may be an increase in seizures. If seizures have been completely controlled or have occurred only very rarely (e.g. once a year), the chance of an increase in seizures during pregnancy is less than if seizures had been frequent before the pregnancy. There is some evidence that an increase in seizures during pregnancy is less likely in patients with primary generalized epilepsy and more likely in those with partial epilepsy.

An increase in seizures during pregnancy may be due to changes in the body chemistry, changes in blood levels of the drugs, or failure to take the antiepileptic drugs, or because of increased tiredness and loss of sleep.

284 Would my epilepsy be better if I had a baby?

No one should have a baby because they hope it will improve their epilepsy. It is not possible to forecast what effect pregnancy will have on epilepsy. There is no reliable evidence that any type of seizure enables one to predict what will happen, nor is there reliable evidence that what happened in a previous pregnancy will happen in the next one.

285 Can I stop my drugs if I want to become pregnant?

It is very unwise to stop medication before deciding to become pregnant because of the risk of seizures, which may harm the mother and the unborn child. (See question 286.)

286 Should I stop my tablets now I am pregnant?

All doctors who specialize in the treatment of epilepsy are agreed that antiepileptic drugs should continue to be taken during pregnancy, because of the risk to the baby is greater if drugs are stopped and the mother has a seizure. Since damage to the baby may occur as early as the first month of pregnancy, often before the mother even knows that she is pregnant, the only way of offering protection would be to stop all drugs before deciding to become pregnant. This may be possible in very special circumstances, with certain drugs and if the seizures are extremely mild and very infrequent, but you must get specialist advice.

Breast feeding is very good for the baby and there is so little of the mother's antiepileptic drug in the milk that it will not harm the baby.

287   Can I take drugs when I am pregnant?

It is important to continue taking drugs during pregnancy. (See question 286 and 289.)

288   If I am pregnant, will my child be born handicapped?

The chance of any mother having an abnormal baby is between 27 and 57 in every 1000 babies. It is known that mothers who have epilepsy are more likely to have an abnormal baby, the risk being twice as high as that in women who do not have epilepsy. Mothers with epilepsy who take antiepileptic drugs are more likely to have an abnormal baby than those with epilepsy who do not take these drugs. What this means is that abnormalities may be due in part to inheritance and in part to the drugs, though no particular drug has yet been proved to produce any particular abnormality.

Abnormalities in babies may be very slight, e.g. unusual shape of the ears or fingernails, or be more important like heart abnormalities, cleft palate or hare-lip, abnormality of the bones or of the nervous system. The minor abnormalities are not serious and do not affect the baby's life. Many, if not most, of the abnormalities can be treated successfully.

Some of the more severe, but rare, abnormalities can be diagnosed early in pregnancy and the mother can therefore be offered an abortion.

289 Will the dose of my drugs need to be altered during my pregnancy?

Pregnancy may alter the chemistry and working of the body and therefore the amount of drugs in the blood may alter, and the mother may therefore need to take a higher dose in order to remain free from seizures. Measurement of the amount of drug in the blood will help the doctor to decide whether changes in medication are needed.

Practical information

Allowances

290 Am I entitled to free prescriptions?

People with epilepsy who require continuous antiepileptic treatment are exempt from prescription charges.

291 How do I obtain free prescriptions?

A leaflet, P11, should be obtained from the post office or social security office. Form C should be completed and then sent to your family doctor.

292 How do I get an attendance allowance?

In order to qualify, an adult or child must be so severely disabled, either physically or mentally, that they require constant attendance to bodily needs and/or continual supervision by another person through the day and night in order to avoid substantial danger to themselves or others. The individual concerned must have been in need of care for 6 months but may claim before the 6 months is up.

There are many additional conditions that must be satisfied, but those outlined above are the main ones.

For detailed information and instructions on how to claim, leaflet N1 205 should be obtained from any social security office and returned to the local social security office.

293   How do I get a mobility allowance?

In order to qualify for the first time the applicant must be aged 5 or over, and not yet have reached the 66th birthday. Once he or she has qualified for the allowance, it can be kept until the individual is 75. Whatever the disability, the applicant must be unable, or virtually unable, to walk because of a physical condition, and be likely to remain so for at least a year. Applicants must be resident in the United Kingdom, and must have been resident in the United Kingdom for at least 12 out of the past 18 months.

In order to claim, leaflet N1 211 should be obtained from a social security office. The claim form attached to it should be filled in, and sent to the address given in Blackpool. Further information on the mobility allowance will be found in the Disability Rights Handbook available from The Disability Alliance, 21 Star Street, London W2 1QB.

294   How do I obtain concessionary travel?

Applicants should get in touch with their local Department of Social Services if they wish to obtain concessionary travel on public road transport. The 1948 National Assistance Act contained clauses referring to transport for disabled people, as also does the 1969 Chronically Sick and Disabled Persons Act. Local authorities are empowered (but not compelled) to provide the means for concessionary travel.

In addition, British Rail has a half-rate travel Railcard for people with disabilities, although the scheme is limited to certain categories of disability. Details of this and other concessions that British Rail offers can be found in a leaflet available from your local British Rail station, or from British Railways Board (Central Publicity Unit), Mulberry House, Marylebone, London NW1.

Holidays

295   Are there any holiday facilities for adults or children with epilepsy?

There should be no need for most people with epilepsy to take segregated holidays. The British Epilepsy Association and its fellow associations have lists of holiday accommodation in hotels, boarding houses and self-catering establishments, in all part of the United Kingdom, where people with epilepsy are welcomed. Special agencies can provide holidays for children with epilepsy which are shared with other handicapped children and able-bodied children also.

It may sometimes be necessary for adults with epilepsy to take supervised group holidays, and on these occasions a hotel is booked for 1 or 2 weeks for the exclusive use of the party. Holidays of this kind are organized by the Epilepsy Centres or by volunteers working for the various epilepsy associations.

Where an individual's financial situation makes payment for a holiday difficult, sponsorship or grants may be available. Further details of all the alternatives listed here are obtainable from the British Epilepsy Association and other epilepsy associations.

296 What activities can my child do in the holidays?

Children with epilepsy on holiday (or at home) can take part in most activities, although precautions and supervision will be necessary in some activities. Most sports can be undertaken, as can swimming, if accompanied by a responsible companion who is also a strong swimmer, and pony-trekking, providing it is a team holiday and the child with epilepsy has adequate head protection.

Cycling is most unwise on public roads, and even on private roads or in parks the child should wear adequate head protection.

It may also be sensible to limit the choice of fairground rides.

The list of activities in which children can be engaged is endless and is a matter for individual decisions in each case.

297 If I go abroad on holiday what do I do about my drugs?

You should take enough drugs to cover the period of your holiday. It is usually possible to obtain enough from your own doctor. If you are going abroad for several months, you may need to get a further supply. Most antiepileptic drugs are easily available in Europe, North America, Australia and the Far East, but there may be difficulty in Africa, India, South East Asia and South America.

If you are taking a large supply of drugs with you, get a letter from your doctor explaining that you have attacks, stating the nature of the drugs and stating that you have to take them daily. This will avoid possible problems with the customs.

298   Can I get medical help abroad?

If you are going to Europe you should ask for a leaflet and application form (SA30) from your local DHSS office. You will have to pay the doctor for medical attendance at the time of the consultation, but you can claim the money back later. However, you would be well advised to take out full insurance cover and this is essential if you are going outside Europe. If you have to be brought home by air ambulance it is very expensive, so make sure that your insurance covers this possibility.

299   Is it safe and can I travel by air?

You can travel by air and it is safe to do so. If your epilepsy is not completely controlled you should consider informing a member of the cabin crew.

300   If I fly long distances will time changes affect my taking of drugs?

Since most drugs can be taken once or twice daily, because they last long enough in the body, it is extremely unlikely that long-distance flights covering many time zones, would affect the taking of antiepileptic drugs.

301   Will jet lag affect my epilepsy?

It is possible that jet lag could affect epilepsy, because jet lag affects the body's circadian rhythm (daily changes throughout 24 hours). However, if there is going to be any affect on the epilepsy it is much more likely to be due to prolonged loss of sleep.

Insurance

302   Can I get car insurance without the premium being loaded?

Not every insurance company applies the same standard. Higher premiums are a harsh reality because, from the insurer's point of view, the risk is greater than normal. The British Epilepsy Association can help with names of those insurance companies who are prepared to issue a policy. Information may be obtained from any of the Association's offices.

303   Can I obtain life insurance without premium loading?

Life insurance is underwritten individually, one of the factors being the severity of the epilepsy. However, a number of insurance companies take a sympathetic and liberal attitude towards those whose lives are impaired or handicapped, and it may be possible to obtain life insurance at only a small extra premium over the normal rate.

Further information as to those companies who will offer life insurance is available from any office of the British Epilepsy Association.

Understanding epilepsy

304   People have a lot of funny ideas about epilepsy — is this common?

People all over the world have funny ideas about epilepsy. This is mainly because a tonic-clonic seizure is frightening to see, and comes without warning, so that someone is normal one moment and then is suddenly struck down. A seizure may therefore be thought to be something to do with the devil or an evil spirit. It is like dying and then reliving, so it is magical. Like insanity, it is difficult to understand and many people believe that epilepsy and insanity are the same, which is quite untrue. Any seizure is so strange, that it is impossible to explain and therefore arouses fear.

Public attitudes are changing, but it is a slow progress. A great many people have no real knowledge of what epilepsy is and is not, and there is an urgent need for more education about epilepsy. The work is currently undertaken by the various epilepsy associations, and it is largely due to their efforts that some improvement in public attitudes has taken place. Nevertheless, there is still a long way to go.

305   Why don't more people understand about epilepsy?

Principally because information is not generally available. Although people may be aware to a certain extent that epilepsy exists, understanding epilepsy means that you have to be prepared to listen, learn and probably change your previous ideas; not everyone is willing to do this.

306   Why am I made to feel different from other people just because I have an occasional fit?

Many people do not understand about epilepsy. Many think that epilepsy just means having a big fit and falling to the ground. Such a seizure is certainly frightening to see, and difficult to understand, and the onlooker may be horrified and feel inadequate and unable to deal with the situation. People who are ignorant are likely to be frightened as well as prejudiced and this affects their attitude, as a result of which they will think that anybody with epilepsy must be 'different'.

307   My parents seem afraid to talk about my epilepsy — why is this?

For many years there has been a great deal of ignorance about epilepsy. Previous generations felt that epilepsy was something shameful and parents may feel that it is their fault that their child has epilepsy. Ignorance leads to fear, and a wish to ignore things or escape from reality — 'don't lets talk about it, lets forget it, it may go away'. Parents with children who have epilepsy are often afraid to discuss epilepsy because they fear (sometimes with justification) the reaction of their friends and neighbours. Will their child be shunned or teased? Sometimes parents will not talk about the child's epilepsy because they are worried that it is due to someone in the father's family or perhaps someone in the mother's family, and these irrational anxieties mean that they keep things to themselves. Sometimes parents worry that if their child knows exactly what happens to them in a fit they will be upset about it.

308 Why does my doctor know so little about epilepsy?

In general, medical students often receive little or no proper teaching about epilepsy, though the amount of teaching has increased in some medical schools in recent years.

A general practitioner has to have a very wide knowledge of all aspects of medicine, so he cannot be expected to be an expert on all conditions. This is why there are hospital specialists, who know 'more and more about less and less'. Most family doctors will have very few (less than 15) patients with epilepsy in their practice.

309 Why don't more doctors know more about epilepsy?

Partly because of lack of training, but partly because each doctor has only relatively few patients with epilepsy. In recent years there have been an increasing number of talks and lectures for general practitioners on epilepsy and an increasing amount of information has been made available by the pharmaceutical firms.

310 What books about epilepsy should I read?

From the many excellent publications, the following titles are of those books that deal with epilepsy generally, as opposed to those that refer only to specific aspects:

1 'Understanding Epilepsy' (second edition) by George Burden and Peter H Schurr, Granada Publishing Limited, Frogmore, St Albans, Herts W1R 4BP.
2 'About Epilepsy' by Donald Scott, Duckworth, The Old Piano Factory, 43 Gloucester Crescent, London NW1 7DY.
3 'Epilepsy Explained' by M V Laidlaw, John Laidlaw, Churchill Livingstone, Robert Stevenson House, 1–3 Baxter's Place, Leith Walk, Edinburgh EH1 3AF.

4   'The Epilepsy Handbook' by Shelagh McGovern,
Sheldon Press, SPCK, Marylebone Road, London NW1
4DU.
5   'Epilepsy — The Facts' by Anthony Hopkins, Oxford
University Press, Walton Street, Oxford OX2 6DP.

A work of fiction by Helen Young entitled 'What difference
does it make Danny?' is interesting reading for children, and
the book is beautifully illustrated. The publishers are Andre
Deutsch, 105 Great Russell Street, London WC1.

311   Can you catch epilepsy? Is it infectious?

Epilepsy is neither catching nor infectious, though it is
believed to be so in many Third World countries.

*312   Why must the word epilepsy be used? Isn't there a less
emotive word?*

When the alternatives to 'epilepsy' are examined, most are
unsatisfactory. Dizzy spells, funny 'do's', 'queer turns',
'convulsions'. None of these terms accurately portray the
condition of epilepsy; for one thing not all epileptic fits are
convulsive. The most acceptable is the American term
'seizure disorder'.
    The trouble with epilepsy is that it has been around for too
long, and historically has had a 'bad press'. Nevertheless,
there has been an improvement in attitudes and the word
'epilepsy' is perhaps slightly less emotive now than it was as
recently as 10 years ago.

*313   Is it right to expect normal children in the family to
have their lives centred around a handicapped sibling?*

No. It would certainly be wrong if a child with a handicap
became the pivot in the family around which everyone else
revolved, especially brothers and sisters. Epilepsy is not
generally considered to be a handicap in the accepted sense
of the word, and the occasional seizure is no reason for
setting the child apart from the family and allowing his
needs to always take priority. The parents should do as much
as they can to explain the nature of the epilepsy to the other

children, and if the attitude of the parents to their child with epilepsy is a balanced one, then that of brothers and sisters is likely to be the same. There is always a certain amount of jealousy and competition for affection amongst normal children in any healthy family. Differences of age, intellect and personality no doubt contribute to this situation. Inevitably parents will have a 'favourite' amongst their children. This is the way family life is lived. But to expect the brothers and sisters of a child with epilepsy to continually defer to the child, to have their routine governed by that child's epilepsy is quite unfair, not only to the other children but also to the child with epilepsy.

5

The Future

Research

314 Why aren't there more new drugs?

Because it costs drug firms millions of pounds to find and
test an entirely new drug, and the chance of getting back all
this money is not great if the drug is for epilepsy compared
with drugs for heart disorder, arthritis, cancer etc. If we can
really find out why seizures occur it should be easier to
produce a suitable drug to control them.

315 Is there any research throwing light on epilepsy?

Research into epilepsy is continuing all the time, but
research into how the brain works is very difficult. Apart
from this basic research, recent and continuing research has
involved the following aspects:

1   The mechanism of action of antiepileptic drugs.
2   The effect of drugs on learning.
3   The interaction of drugs.
4   The influence of epilepsy and drugs on the unborn child.
5   The role of hormones in epilepsy.
6   The value of a new investigation — Positron Emission
    Computed Tomography. This is a sort of super CT scan
    that also gives information about the function of the
    brain.

7   The attitudes of people with epilepsy to themselves, and that of the general population to those with epilepsy.

Each year there are hundreds of scientific papers about epilepsy.

316   Is the lack of progress due to shortage of money or the complexity of the subject?

Lack of progress is due to shortage of money and the complexity of the subject. Much research nowadays depends on money from charities or from drug companies, though funds are received from the Medical Research Council and various medical trusts.

Appendices

Epilepsy organizations world wide

All addresses are correct at time of going to press.
Information can be obtained from the following lay organizations:

1   **Australia**
 a. National Epilepsy Association of Australia, P.O. Box 554, Lilydale, VIC. 3140 Australia.
 b. Epilepsy Foundation of Victoria, 818–822 Burke Road, Camberwell, VIC. 3124 Australia.
 c. Epilepsy Association of Queensland, Room 438, Penney's Buildings, 210 Queen Street, Brisbane, QLD. 4000 Australia.
 d. West Australian Epilepsy Association (Inc.), 14 Bagot Road, Subiaco, W.A. 6008 Australia.
 e. Epileptic Welfare Association (N.S.W.), P.O. Box 521, Pennant Hills, N.S.W. 2120 Australia.
 f. Epilepsy Association of S.A. Inc., P.O. Box 596, Prospect East, S.A. 5082, Australia.
 g. Epilepsy Association of Tasmania Inc., P.O. Box 421, Sandy Bay, TAS. 7005, Australia.

h. Epilepsy Association of the A.C.T. Inc., 22 Rich Place, Higgins, A.C.T. 2615, Australia.

2 **Canada** (there is no national association)
   a. Epilepsy Canada, 2145 Lakeshore, Dorval, Quebec H9S 2G4.
   b. Edmonton Epilepsy Association, 308–10012 Jasper Avenue, Edmonton, Alberta T5J 1R7.
   c. British Colombia Epilepsy Association, 1195 West 8th Avenue, Vancouver, B.C. V6H 1C5.
   d. Epilepsy Association of Calgary, 2422 5th Avenue N.W., Calgary, Alberta T2N 0TZ.
   e. Epilepsy Ontario – Mid West Region, 267 Dundas Street, Suite 39, London, Ontario N6A 1H2.
   f. Metro Toronto, 214 King Street West, Suite 214, Toronto, Ontario M5H 1K4.

3 **Denmark**
Dansk Epilepsiforening, Admiralgade 15, 1066 Copenhagen K.

4 **India**
The Indian Epilepsy Association, 251 Dr. D. Naoroji Road, Fort, Bombay 400001.

5 **The Netherlands**
Epilepsie Voreniging Nederland, Koningsblaan 19, 3583 Utrecht.

6 **New Zealand**
New Zealand Epilepsy Association, P.O. Box 683, Hamilton.

7 **South Africa**
South African National Epilepsy League, P.O. Box 4197, 201–203 Barclays Bank Building, Church Square, Pretoria.

8 **U.S.A.**
Epilepsy Foundation of America, Suite 406, 4351 Garden City Drive, Landover, Maryland 20785.

For information about other worldwide organizations not included in the previous list, contact the British Epilepsy Association.

The International League Against Epilepsy is primarily a medical or professional organization, and information may be obtained from branches (or chapters) in the following countries:

1 **Argentina**
Liga Argentina Contra la Epilepsia, Tucuman 3261, 1189 Buenos Aires.

2 **Austria**
The Chapter of ILAE in Austria, Dr. K. Patysky, Lazarettgasse 14, A — 1090 Vienna.

3 **Bolivia**
The Chapter of ILAE in Bolivia, Dr. Mario Michel Zamora, Casilla 3370, La Paz.

4 **Brazil**
Liga Brasileira de Epilepsia, c/o Dr. Amauri Batista da Silva, SQS 307 B.D.Ap. 303–70354, Brasilia, D.F.

5 **Canada**
Canadian League Against Epilepsy, Henry Dunn, M.B., F.R.C.P., F.R.C.P.(C)., Pediatric Neurology, Health Center for Children, 715 West 12th Avenue, Vancouver B.C. V5Z 1 M9.

6 **Chile**
Liga Chilena contra la Epilepsia, P.O. Box 150, Viña del Mar, Chile.

7 **Columbia**
Liga Central contra la Epilepsia, Dr. Carlos Medina-Malo, Segretario Ejecutivo, Apartado Aéreo 057751, Bogotà. D.E.

8 **Czechoslovakia**
Czechoslovak League Against Epilepsy, Prof. Ivan Lesny, V. Uvalu 84, 15006 Praha 5, Motol.

9 **Denmark**
Danish Epilepsy Society, Dr. Birthe Pedersen, Hon. Secretary, Røhrholmsgade 22, 5/th, DK — 1352 Copenhagen K.

10 **Dominican Republic**
Sociedad Dominicana contra la Epilepsia, Dr. Julio
Oscar Tejada Jaquez, The Amado Garcia Querrero No.
233, Santo Domingo.

11 **France**
Ligue Francaise contre l'Epilepsie, c/o Dr. Paul Favel,
Etablissement Médical de la Teppe, 26600 Tain-L'Her-
mitage.

12 **Finland**
Finnish Epilepsy Association, Dr. Ulrich Tackee,
Secretary-General, Dept. of Neurology, University of
Kuopio, 70210 Kuopio 21.

13 **West Germany**
Prof. Dr. med. R. Kruse, Südwestdeutsches Epilep-
siezentrum Kehl, 7640 Kehl-Kork.

14 **East Germany**
The Chapter of ILAE in East Germany, c/o Prof. Dr.
Sc.Med.G. Rabending, Vorz. der Gesellschaft für
Neuroelektro-diagnostik der DDR, Direktor der
Nervenklinik der Ernst-Moritz-Arndt-Universität, DDR
— 22 Greifswald.

15 **Great Britain**
The Chapter of ILAE British Branch, Dr. David
Chadwick, Honorary Secretary, Department of
Neurology, Walton Hospital, Liverpool.

16 **Israel**
The Israel League Against Epilepsy, Dr. Jehudit
Manelis, Secretary, P.O. Box 9611, Haifa.

17 **Italy**
Lega Italiana contro l'Epilessia, Prof. C. Alberto
Tassinari, Presidente, Via U. Foscolo, 7, 40123 Bologna.

18 **Japan**
The Japanese Epilepsy Society, Dr. Toyoji Wada,
National Musashi Research Institute for Mental and
Nervous Diseases, 2620 Ogawa-Higashi, Kodaira (MZ
187), Tokyo.

19 **Mexico**
Mexican League Against Epilepsy, Dr. Teodoro Flores-Rodriguez, Insurgentes Sur. No. 3877, Col. La Fama, Deleg. Tlalpan, 14410 Mexico, D.F.

20 **The Netherlands**
The Chapter of ILAE in The Netherlands, Dr. Harry Meinardi, delegate, Instituut voor Epilepsiebestrijding, Achterweg 5, 2103 SW Heemstede.

21 **Norway**
The Chapter of ILAE in Norway, Dr. Wollert Krohn, Statens Center for Epilepsi, P.O. Box 900, 1301 Sandvika.

22 **Poland**
The Chapter of ILAE in Poland, Dr. Jerzy Majkowski, Lindleya 4, 02-005 Warsawa, Poland.

23 **Spain**
Liga Española contra la Epilepsia, Dr. J. Villa-Bado, President, Platon 3,3,1 Barcelona 2.

24 **Sweden**
The Chapter of ILAE in Sweden, c/o Dr. Karl-Axel Melin, 13 Bagargrand, 2 — 123 54 Farsta.

25 **Switzerland**
The Chapter of ILAE in Switzerland, c/o Mrs. Vreni Koeppel, Pro Infirmis, Postfach 129, 8032 Zurich.

26 **U.S.A.**
The American Epilepsy Society, Suite 304, Prof. Building, 179 Allyn Street, Hartford, CT 06103.

27 **Uruguay**
Liga Uruguaya contra la Epilepsia, Dra. Edith Gerstle de Pasquet, Instituto de Neurologia, P.2, Hospital de Clinicas, Montevideo, Uruguay.

Index

THE HEART DISEASE REFERENCE BOOK. Direct and Clear Answers to Everyone's Questions

by Alan Mackintosh, MA, MD, MRCP

Raises all the questions everyone wants to ask and answers them as accurately as current knowledge permits.

This invaluable reference book provides a full account of heart disease, symptoms, diagnosis, treatment and prevention. Heart disease is the commonest fatal illness in the westernized world, and is partly preventable. This book provides information on policy and social pressures as well as medical fact.

* Clear question-and-answer format allows easy and quick reference.
* Medical concepts are explained in a straightforward and direct manner.
* The most common types of heart disease are detailed — causes, symptoms, diagnostic methods, treatment and rehabilitation.
* Preventive actions are discussed in detail.
* Offers advice and support for family members and friends of the heart patient.

Health Reference Series
0 06 318297 1 Paper 224pp approx
8¼" × 6" £3.95 September 1984

The
Heart
Disease
Reference
Book Alan Mackintosh

DIRECT AND
CLEAR ANSWERS
TO EVERYONE'S
QUESTIONS

THE ANOREXIA NERVOSA REFERENCE BOOK.
Direct and Clear Answers to Everyone's Questions

by Roger Slade

Raises all the questions everyone wants to ask and answers them as accurately as current knowledge permits.

There are real difficulties in understanding anorexia nervosa and in helping the anorexic to overcome the condition. *The Anorexia Nervosa Reference Book* offers information and advice about this problem.

* Clear question-and-answer format allows easy and quick reference.
* Medical and psychological concepts are explained in a straightforward and direct manner.
* Advice and support are offered to the anorexic and the family.
* Explains the physiological aspects of anorexia.
* Outlines the psychological consequences of starvation.
* Relates anorexia to family and social pressures.

Health Reference Series
0 06 318296 3 Paper 224pp approx
8¼" × 6" £3.95 September 1984

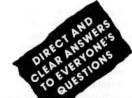

The
Anorexia
Nervosa
Reference
Book   Roger Slade

DIRECT AND CLEAR ANSWERS TO EVERYONE'S QUESTIONS

THE CANCER REFERENCE BOOK.
Direct and Clear Answers to Everyone's Questions

by Paul Levitt and Elissa Guralnick with A. Robert Kagan and Harvey Gilbert

Raises all the questions everyone wants to ask and answers them as accurately as current knowledge permits.

This reference book covers a range of subjects from what cancer is, how it begins and spreads, to methods of treatment (surgery, chemo- and radiotherapy) and current research.

* The clear question-and-answer format allows easy and quick reference.
* Details 21 most common types of cancer, describing the organ; how the cancer affects it; symptoms diagnosis; treatment; possible side effects of treatment, prognosis; geographical, age, occupational patterns; and specific causes.
* Defines the important terms.
* Provides a list of cancer centres throughout the world.
* Offers advice and support in terminal care, for the patient and the family.
* Surveys current cancer research.
* Gives information about prevention and dietary advice.
* Explodes some of the myths about unproven cancer treatments.

Health Reference Series
0 06 318230 0 Paper 224pp 8¼" × 6"
£3.95 September 1984

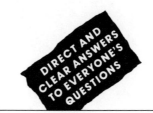

The
Cancer
Reference
Book

Paul M. Levitt and
Elissa S. Guralnick

with Dr A Robert Kagan and Dr Harvey Gilbert

DIRECT AND CLEAR ANSWERS TO EVERYONE'S QUESTIONS